COVER

the principles and art of para-medical skin camouflage

Elizabeth Allen

authorHOUSE®

AuthorHouse™ UK
1663 Liberty Drive
Bloomington, IN 47403 USA
www.authorhouse.co.uk
Phone: 0800.197.4150

First published by AuthorHouse 2010
Second edition published by AuthorHouse 2015

Published by AuthorHouse 08/11/2015

ISBN: 978-1-4520-6603-5 (sc)

Print information available on the last page.

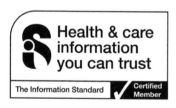

Cover, the principles and art of para-medical skin camouflage
text has gained Plain English Campaign 'Approved by' logo
and meets the Information Standard criteria,
which confirms that BASC is a producer of high quality,
reliable health and social care information

This book is printed on acid-free paper.

British Association of Skin Camouflage
website www.skin-camouflage.net
Registered Charity in England & Wales (No. 1123059)
Scottish Registered Charity (No. SC045283)

BASC is a company limited by guarantee, registered in England & Wales No. 06156591
Registered Office: GHP Legal 26-30 Grosvenor Road Wrexham LL11 1BU (ref JM)

acknowledgements and credits

the author is especially grateful to those who so kindly volunteered their time and expertise to contribute and to comment on the text of this handbook (note not all listed participated in revisions for the 2015 reprint),
Mr Tim Goodacre MSc MB BS FRCS
– Senior Clinical Lecturer in the Nuffield Department of Surgery, University of Oxford
  and Consultant Plastic Surgeon, Radcliffe Infirmary, Oxford
James Partridge OBE
– Founder and Chief Executive of *Changing Faces*
Christine Piff
– Founder of *Let's Face It*

Cosmetic Chemist	Jo Larner MSc SCSDip CSci CChem MRSC
Dermatology	Professor Andrew Wright B.Med.Sci(Hons) LRCP MRCS MBCHB FRCP
Dermatology	Dr Catherine Hardman MB BS MRCP
Experimental Chemist	Lynne Ashton
LASER & IPL	Dr Samantha Hills PhD (Clinical and training Manager, Lynton Lasers)
Ophthalmology	Mr Stewart Armstrong MRCP FRCS FRC.Ophth DO
Plastic Surgery	Ms Beryl De Souza FRCS MPhil MBBS BSc(Hons)
Plastic Surgery	Mr Tim Goodacre MSc MB BS FRCS
Plastic Surgery	Mr Richard Price MD FRCS(Plast)
Psychology	Dr Linda Papadopoulos CPsychol CSci AFBPsS
A-Z of Conditions	the Patient Support Groups associated with the condition

Skin Camouflage - a potted history
the historical information on Joyce Allsworth could not have been achieved without kind assistance from BASC's Jane Goulding and Thelma Giles; Ruth Russell and Doreen St John Cooper (Red Cross); The Guinea Pig Club and Bond McIndoe Museum at Queen Victoria Hospital East Grinstead; and the information supplied by the camouflage and cosmetic companies mentioned.

for their patience and sharing their advice and experience on written sections, the author would like to thank BASC past and present committee members,
Dawn Cragg, MBE (Medical Tattooing), Sally-Jane Dawson (Beauty Therapy), Gillian Hart (IPL and LASER), Liz Hawkins (Plastic Surgery Nursing), Sheila Heaviside (Nails), Diane Jones (Prosthetics), Jules Stevenson (Make-up), Kim Davies (Plastic Surgery Nursing), Jane Goulding (ingredients definition), Sharon Lane and Mary Thorp (editorial team), Jami Easom and Maggie Richards (for organising photographic sessions in London). We also thank Dawn Forshaw (Finishing Touches) and all the wonderful people who kindly permitted us to use their image; and to Helen Martins who so patiently edited the text and transferred the concept of camouflage into this handbook

we would like to thank the following photographers for the BASC copyrighted material in this book,
photograph numbers prefix 01 by Paul at Dream Media, Chester
photograph numbers prefix 02 by Dave Sellens, ABPPA, London
photograph numbers prefix 03 by Darren Richards, Chester
photograph numbers prefix 04 by Richard Alli
our gratitude for all other photographs which are reproduced with kind courtesy by BASC members, patients, patient support groups and organisations (copyright acknowledged).

a special acknowledgement goes to BASC ex-chair Sheila Dutch
without whom this project would never have got off the ground

our debt of gratitude,
we remain grateful to Joyce Allsworth for her inspirational work

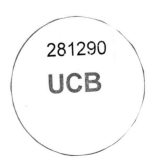

I'M STILL ME

What a lovely child they said,
Now they look away instead

Oh, my, isn't she pretty,
Now they say "Oh what a pity."

Is it me they talk about?
They think I'm deaf, so they shout!
because I'm scarred, I've been burned
and through my pain I have learned
that because I no longer look the same,
deep within me burns the pain.

Not through memories of before,
when I was different, and much more
but because I'm made to feel ashamed
it feels as if I should be blamed
for looking as I do today
for making others turn away.

But no more shall I feel shy,
As they stare and pass me by.

I shall hold my head for all to see,
It's they who've changed – I'm still me!

poem by Jaimi
reproduced with kind permission of Christine Piff, Let's Face It *'Children's Faces'*

contents

foreword

the crucial role of skin camouflage

The use of skin camouflage methods of therapy for those with non-infectious skin conditions and scarring offers remarkable benefits to holistic patient care. However, in recent years it has been somewhat overshadowed by the considerable publicity given to new 'high tech' surgical procedures which have developed within surgical science. Skin camouflage, along with a number of other therapeutic disciplines (such as prosthetics), has suffered from not being included in the core teaching of those involved with managing such patients, and especially from a paucity of practical literature on the subject. The absence of any books on camouflage methods alongside the plethora of surgical technical tomes at medical meeting exhibitions is testament to this imbalance.

Being fortunate enough to begin my training in plastic surgery at the beginning of the era of contemporary high tech methods, the senior surgeons to whom I was apprenticed nurtured considerable respect for the wide variety of means to manage disfiguring conditions throughout a patient's lifetime. I thus came into contact with the late Joyce Allsworth at an early stage in my career, and was immediately impressed by the enthusiasm, commitment and highly developed professional skill that she brought to her work. The use of techniques to reduce the visual impact of skin conditions, she added an invaluable tool to the toolbox of care that is brought into use within every consultation. I was unaware at the time of the history that lay behind such work, but was impressed by the way Joyce and her equally skilled and enthusiastic colleagues sought both to refine and pass on their knowledge.

Since that time, many new surgical methods have been developed, to the great benefit of many patients who might otherwise have been subject to multiple staged reconstructive procedures, with less efficacious outcomes. However, these new operations have not always been accompanied by wise judgment in their use. Not infrequently, an enthusiastic and technically adept surgeon leaps to the use of some surgical manoeuvre which, whilst offering something of a 'fix' to a perceived problem, fails to produce an end result which in any way satisfied the patient's concerns overall. Such surgically fixated 'triumphs of technique over reason' are often bad enough on their own. However, they are frequently accompanied by the perception that adjunctive methods such as camouflage are somewhat old fashioned and less valuable. This could not be further from the truth. It is vital that a proper perspective be restored to the management of skin conditions – a perspective which does not nurture the early 21st century belief (in both the public and professional mindset) that there is a surgical-mechanical 'fix' for all ills.

It is with that background that I was delighted to hear of the updating and publication of an entirely new edition of Joyce Allsworth's book, so long out of print and unavailable to a new generation of health carers. Its reappearance is timely, joining a rediscovery of many means of managing problems other than surgery – these more often than not led by nurses, therapists and others outside conventional 'medical' training.

The new work has been superbly rewritten and expanded into a comprehensive, yet readable, guide for all involved in such care. Following the overview of conditions that can be managed and a detailed description of cosmetic methods, the book closes with a valuable and informative history of skin camouflage and its development in the United Kingdom. I have little doubt that exciting new methods lie ahead, and will be built upon the solid foundation outlined in this book. It deserves to be read and used widely, and certainly should be in every library of those caring for those with skin conditions. Thank you Joyce and your successors for this legacy.

Tim Goodacre MSc MB BS FRCS
Senior Clinical Lecturer in the Nuffield Department of Surgery, University of Oxford
and Consultant Plastic Surgeon, Radcliffe Infirmary, Oxford.
Patron to BASC

defining the role of the camouflage practitioner

your role is an important pivot in helping people regain confidence and self-esteem through the simple application of skin camouflage products

defining the role of the camouflage practitioner

The role of the camouflage practitioner is to take people through a skin matching process to identify an acceptable skin colour match and the product best suited to their needs. Once this has been agreed then the appropriate camouflage application technique is taught. Obviously, anyone requesting your camouflage advice is affected and distressed by their image, therefore during the consultation your attitude towards them will be of paramount importance. To paraphrase Sir Archibald McIndoe *"always be 50% medical and 50% psychological"* in your approach because the psychological benefit to a person who has been taught how to successfully apply and manage their skin camouflage cannot be over-emphasised.

We all strive to be socially accepted within our community, but sadly we are also influenced by an image-conscious media to conform to society's narrow definition of beauty. The result is that most people report that at some point they have met with rejection, name-calling, unwarranted comments, intrusive questioning or verbal abuse. People may refrain from consulting their medical advisor believing their condition will be dismissed as "cosmetic" rather than "medical" and that they will be branded as being vain. It has long been acknowledged that mind and body interact upon each other. Although there is no accepted definition of HRQoL (health-related quality of life) it is self evident that when a person is disturbed by some aspect of their appearance then, inevitably, their general health and quality of life will be adversely affected. Without help they can withdraw from employment, domestic and social-sporting activities which in turn may affect the quality of life of their family members. Studies into psychosocial behaviour are well documented – all conclusions indicate that low self-esteem is equally devastating to men, women and children, irrespective of age, nationality, religion and skin classification group. Psychosocial inhibition is also irrespective of whether the problem is immediately visible or hidden by clothing.

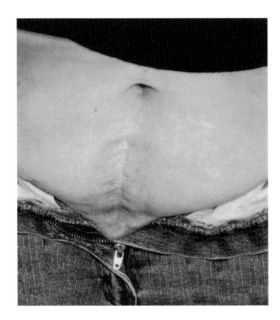 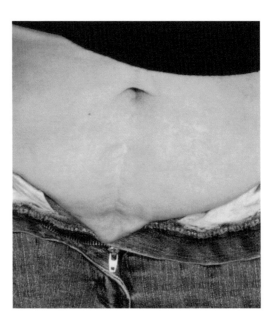

01 psychosocial inhibition is irrespective of size and the condition
being immediately visible or hidden by clothing

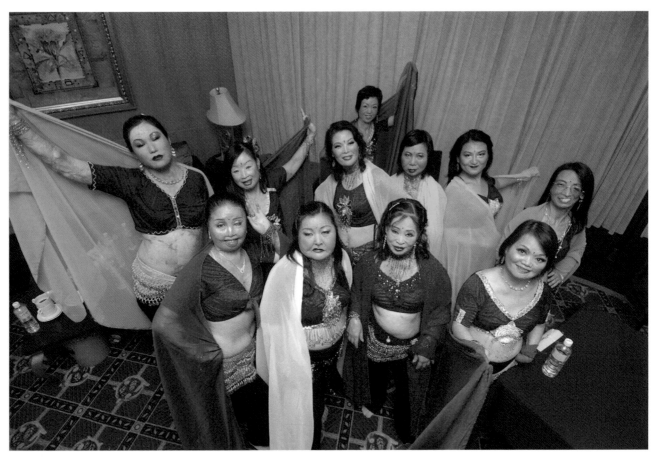

as part of its psychosocial rehabilitation work, the Sunshine Foundation started
a belly- dancing troupe in 2006 composed of ladies with burn scarring.
Skin camouflage is used during public performances to enhance theatrical effect,
but also to highlight the vitality and self-confidence of dancers
comfortable with their body and passionate about their dancing.
© Sunshine Foundation, Taiwan, (BASC Honorary Member)

professional code of conduct and codes of practice

being a professional you will know that dermatoses and scarring have many causes. Some people with congenital disorders may be born with the condition apparent, while for others their hereditary dermatosis can present at a later stage – and that is usually when it is least welcome, particularly during puberty. Many, especially those recently diagnosed, may not have met anyone with the same condition – you can help lessen their isolation by telling them about any local or national groups that can offer additional advice and support. It is helpful to put a folder of useful information in the waiting room for people to browse through.

Those who have imperfections to their skin (whatever the cause) are very aware (sometimes hypersensitive) to body language. Wittingly or unwittingly your actions can suggest an erroneous assumption about their character and personal hygiene. Your approach is crucial; any tendency to show a negative attitude could increase the person's anxiety. All responses should be positive and encouraging, while not agreeing to any unrealistic expectations they may have. It is generally accepted that skin camouflage can be a vital tool during the early stages of someone's rehabilitation and adjustment to an altered image. For others, wearing skin camouflage may need to be considered long-term.

Camouflage products are never called cosmetics or make-up. The term 'skin camouflage' creates no psychological barriers – it is non-exclusive – whereas 'cosmetics' and 'make-up' can create all kinds of anxiety to those who would not normally wear decorative cosmetics. It is axiomatic that if people have a psychological barrier to the terminology used, then they will not come to you for advice. Camouflage is designed to replicate the colours of skin for a para-medical purpose and should not be confused with fashionable beauty aids. The terminology para-medical indicates a supplementary aid which complements the restorative reason for skin camouflage. However there will be occasions when someone requests skin camouflage for an aesthetic, personal and non-medical reason, such as to cover a tattoo during working hours or for a single occasion, for example a wedding.

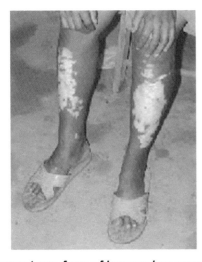

at its onset one form of leprosy has exactly the same appearance as vitiligo. While leprosy is very uncommon in developed countries, it does still exist. When vitiligo is mistaken for leprosy the person often becomes a social outcast, ostracised by their community; in this illustration this happened until the local missionaries were able to source and secure camouflage products for this lady.
© Alida DePase, BASC Member 2158

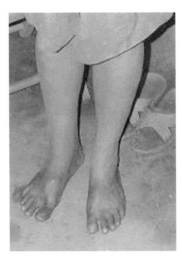

the happy result is that being "cured of leprosy" she is now totally reintegrated within her village life.
© Alida DePase, BASC Member 2158

When you meet someone, walk towards them in a welcoming manner, smile, make eye contact and shake their hand; this will do much to reassure people who have shied away from social contact. Always position yourself next to them. A desk, couch or trolley between you can create a psychological barrier. An initial non-invasive distance of about .75m (2'6") is generally considered the optimum space. If they are accompanied, ask that person to sit on the other side of them and not between you.

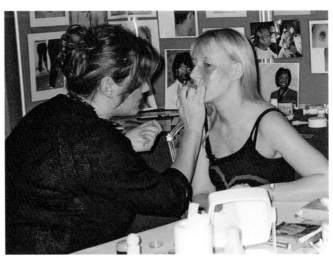

once the person is relaxed, you can then sit or stand closer to them without creating anxiety

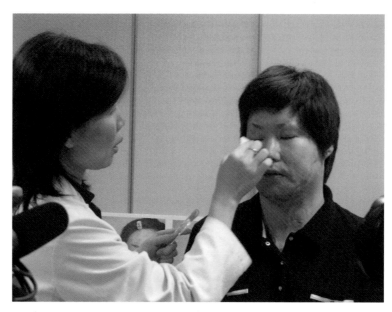

always face the patient for skin camouflage application
Yun-Ju Lin (trained by BASC)
© Sunshine Foundation, Taiwan, (**BASC** Honorary Member)

Learn to really listen to what the person is saying – both spoken and body language. Some may take a while to build up enough confidence to show you what needs camouflaging. If they are very hesitant, explain why camouflage may be helpful and demonstrate its properties on yourself. Your own verbal and body language can do much to relax them. Remember to communicate in everyday speech, explaining any medical and technical terminology used.

You will come across a variety of skin conditions, dermatoses and scarring. In some cases the area needing camouflage will be small but there will be occasions when the skin has been greatly affected. The severity of the condition is not a key factor. What may seem trivial to you is obviously causing them concern – *"Before I judge my neighbour, let me walk a mile in his moccasins"*.
Heinmot Tooyalaket (Chief Joseph) d.1904 of the Nez Percés, Native American

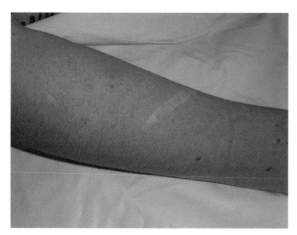

hypopigmentation
© BASC Member 2303

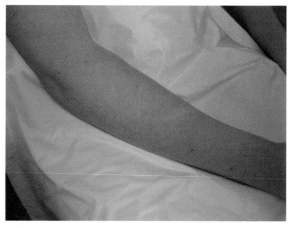

camouflage applied
© BASC Member 2303

In the case of fresh scars, it is desirable to camouflage these as soon as possible, providing the wound is sealed and healed. At this point the appearance is at its worst and the psychological effect is most damaging. With the permission of the doctor, camouflage applied at this early stage can also hide any bruising.

People may present themselves to you without having first consulted their medical advisor; they may be embarrassed or think that asking for camouflage would waste their valuable surgery time. They may also believe that their request would be dismissed, as the condition is not 'life-threatening'. If the person does not want their medical team to know that they are seeking camouflage, then you cannot breach this request. However, you should gently suggest that their medical practitioner be informed to enable records to be updated. They may find that their medical advisor is more receptive than they thought, or possibly that they are totally unaware of camouflage! Many medical professionals are indeed unaware that camouflage is available and will merely advise people that nothing more can be done and that they 'must learn to live with it'. Some may think of camouflage as make-up, or a decorative product suitable only for adult females. This lack of understanding should disappear once camouflage becomes acknowledged as a tool to rehabilitation and included as an option within aftercare treatment plans.

There may be occasions when you must question whether it is advisable to offer skin camouflage. Neither you, nor the person, should self-diagnose, but should anything look suspicious then you must advise the person to seek medical opinion before proceeding with any skin camouflage. Make a note on their file and arrange a future consultation. You must also advise people to seek medical advice if any changes take place to the area requiring camouflage (especially a mole) and to discontinue their camouflage until they have received their medical advisor's permission to continue.

If information about the condition was given to you when the appointment was made (or in a letter from a medical practitioner) it is essential to allow the person to explain their requirements at the consultation. Even if a condition appears apparent to you, never assume that is the reason - the particular problem may not be immediately visible. Indeed, anything obvious to you may NOT prove to be the one that is worrying them. Jumping to conclusions can lead to a wrong assessment being made: this can cause embarrassment to both of you and can also cause considerable harm by drawing attention to something which the person readily accepts as part of their image.

Although **you** may be curious to know the history of the scar, bruise or dermatosis, do not make the person feel they are obliged to tell you. If they want you to know, they will volunteer information. Many people agree that it is their emotional association and not the actual scar or dermatosis which causes greater distress. Unless it is vital information that would affect the camouflage application, the consultation should not be intrusive.

I keep six honest serving-men,
(They taught me all I knew) :
Their names are What and Why and When and How and Where and Who
Rudyard Kipling, *Just So Verses - The Elephant's Child*

Although these words may have served Kipling they are **not** essential questions you need to ask. Respect people's privacy and do not allow **your** curiosity to re-open **their** psychological wounds. This important rule also applies to decorative tattoos, especially any medical marking made by Radiographers.

It is vital that everyone is given equal professionalism and empathy. Whilst it is a natural human temptation to offer unsolicited advice – it would be totally unethical to do so. There is a temptation to make an encouraging comment, such as "what a nicely healed scar" – such an observation, although well intended, can create more harm than good. The person will have a psychological association to the area requiring camouflage – and it matters not, to them, how you perceive their problem!

Whilst you should never dismiss anyone's problem as being insignificant it is equally important you do not suggest or agree that they have an insurmountable problem. However, you may come across a patient with dysmorphophobia (body dysmorphia is a disorder where they have an obsessive fear that part or all of them is repulsive, or may become so). You may also see someone who has undergone treatment which has much improved their scar or dermatosis but, to their eyes, the problem is just as great as it was before, or even greater. For such patients, camouflage may play little part until their psychiatric condition is resolved, but can be a significant part of their overall treatment.

Camouflage can play a vital role in the recovery of people who self-harm as their injuries are not so apparent once camouflaged. There is also some therapeutic value when applying camouflage because the person is touching their skin in a benign way. People benefit psychologically from touching their scar or dermatosis – it gets them used to looking and handling their altered image and can do much to help them through the stages of grief outlined in Chapter 11.

It is absolutely fundamental that people are involved in selecting products and fully understand by the end of the session how to self-apply their camouflage, how to maintain it during wear and removal procedures. If a child or someone who will rely on another person to apply the camouflage, it is still important to talk to and to involve them – not just the accompanying person. Although you will need to ensure that the parent or carer understands everything, you you must include the person at every stage. You may find that members of some cultures do not allow non-family members or people outside their religion to touch them directly; in those instances you will need to make sure the person is accompanied by someone who can perform the camouflage process under your direction.

To avoid any accusation of abuse, it may be inappropriate for you to work directly on a member of the opposite sex, especially when applying camouflage to sensitive areas of the body. In this case you will need to explain that a third party needs to be present, but that they will not take an active part in the camouflage consultation.

This also applies when offering camouflage to a minor, when the accompanying adult should remain in the room. The parent or guardian may be required to give signed consent to camouflage application for minors. It is also necessary to check relevant legislation to ensure you have the appropriate consent to work with minors. Children under the age of two have little, if any, sense of their identity but however young any rejection and negativity to their image can have a long-term psychological effect. BASC does not recommend the use of camouflage products on very young children. However, there may be occasions when it could be acceptable – for example, to conceal a strawberry birthmark (which would not be present later in life) for a single event such as an important family occasion or photograph. On these occasions you must apply common sense and be cautious that your actions are not masking child abuse.

No one, especially children, should be made to feel that they must use camouflage. However, a child may be well adjusted to their image until puberty (or when they become more influenced by the media) or when moving from a small, local primary to a large secondary school where the majority of their new peers are strangers.

You should always be honest when discussing outcomes. Sometimes a person will also ask your opinion on available treatments and products which might improve the condition of their skin. Maybe you are qualified to provide additional treatments, such as electrolysis on a flap, or at least be able to advise which local beauty therapist can provide that service. The media can be misleading and frequently give the impression that a product or treatment is readily available when, in fact, it is still undergoing clinical trials and may not be available for some considerable time. People will try anything to "make it better" and here are some suggested responses to questions you may be asked,

food supplements : will they improve and cure my problem?

EU law does permit certain health claims to be made where these can be scientifically substantiated, for example, claims which relate to the role of a nutrient or other substance in growth, development and the functions of the body. However, the EU directive stipulates that the labelling, presentation and advertising must not attribute to food and food supplements the properties to prevent, treat or cure a human disease. The moment a named medical condition is attached to any product or claim, then it falls under the legislation associated with the licence and sale of drugs.

IPL and LASER treatments : where should I go for advice?

at the time of going to print, current continuation of regulation and registration of LASER (Light Amplification by Stimulated Emission of Radiation) and IPL (Intense Pulsed Light) based devices is under review. We suggest the person confirm that the operator and clinic have fully complied with the Insurance and required Protocols (including patch tests) before undergoing treatment. People are also advised to seek opinion from their doctor before undergoing any IPL or LASER treatment and, most importantly, comply with contraindications before and throughout the course of treatment.

purchases and treatments

before entering into any sale (including those from the internet) everyone should always ensure that the product and equipment is fit for purpose, is licenced for sale and complies with EU legislation, and that the purveyor has the required qualifications to perform the treatment. The old adage "if it sounds too good to be true…then it probably is" should not be forgotten!

consultations

each new case presents a challenge. Your priority is to establish a rapport, remembering not to make elaborate claims, never promise perfection! It is essential to emphasise that camouflage will not return the texture of the skin to how it was before, but can make the dermatosis or scar less noticeable.

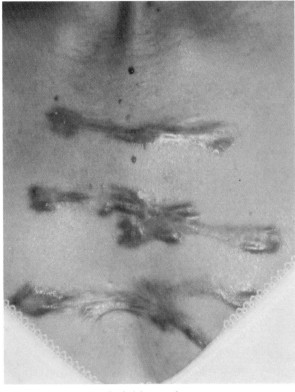

keloid scarring
© BASC Member 1022

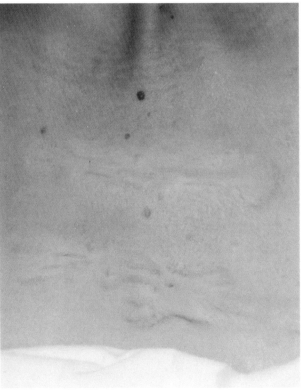

following camouflage application
© BASC Member 1022

Skin camouflage will always achieve a better outcome when the dermatosis and scarring does not create a different structure to the skin.

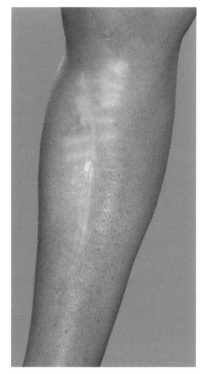 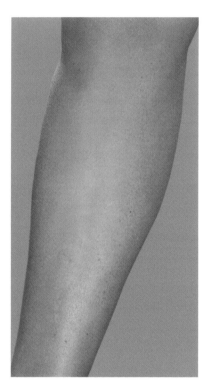

01 road traffic accident scarring,
flat to surrounding skin

01 camouflage applied

Ideally, a half to one hour should be set aside for each consultation. This should allow sufficient time for a nervous person to relax and for you to create an acceptable skin match and, if required, to reproduce any natural characteristics, such as the freckles or beard shadow needed to fully camouflage the area. You need to explain how to apply and remove camouflage and also what toiletries or activities might unwittingly disturb it. The person needs to know the brands and colours used and where they can obtain supplies. People will need a revised skin match consultation when their dermatosis, scar or surrounding skin changes colour.

The consultation must allow time for the person to demonstrate to you that they fully understand the application and removal techniques. At first attempt, some may find the camouflage routine laborious, or apply too much product. You will be thoroughly familiar with the routine of applying and removing camouflage but but the person almost certainly will not. Do encourage them to persevere and practise. The more they use their camouflage, the more expert they will become and it is important to point that out. It is always helpful to give people a procedure guideline to follow (as opposite example).

It may be a workplace requirement or just your civility to contact people a few weeks after their initial consultation to ask if they are experiencing any difficulty in managing their camouflage routine or obtaining supplies. Obviously, a follow-up is not necessary when you have applied the camouflage for a single requirement, such as concealing a bride's tattoo for her wedding.

It is necessary and important for you to keep a record of the camouflage consultation and outcome for future reference, as the example given (page 14). People and their records must be treated in strict confidence and comply with Data Protection Acts, with whom you may be required to register.

Applying your skin camouflage

Step 1
Make sure your hands and the area you are applying camouflage to are clean and dry. Unless necessary, there is no need to apply a skin toner.

Step 2
Hygienically remove enough skin camouflage from its container.

Step 3
Place the camouflage in your palm – this will slightly warm it which makes it quicker to apply.

Mix two colours together in your palm (if we have suggested this to achieve an acceptable skin match).

Step 4
Using the technique we agreed with you, apply the camouflage to the relevant area, trying to avoid the unaffected skin, then blend the edges.

Step 5
Load the powder puff and gently pat and roll the powder over the area. Wait a moment or two for the powder to be absorbed.

Step 6
Carefully brush off any excess powder.

If you need more cover, repeat steps 2 to 6.

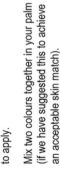

Throw away products once they reach their 'use before' date (see the packaging for more information).

Removing your skin camouflage

The following will quickly remove your camouflage:

★ soap and water
★ soap substitute (cleansing lotions and creams)
★ cosmetic cleansing wipes
★ oil-based products (such as aromatherapy oils)
★ oil-based sun protection
★ moisturisers and emollients

Remove your camouflage each day – this will allow you to apply any skin medication, sun protection and moisturisers. It will also give you the opportunity to inspect your skin for any changes which may need medical attention.

Managing your skin camouflage

Camouflage is waterproof, which means you can swim and enjoy sporting activities. When the camouflage area is wet, let your skin dry naturally if you can. Otherwise, carefully pat it dry, as rubbing it with a towel will remove the camouflage.

Take extra care on areas where the product may rub or wash off (such as back of hands, collar and cuffs).

You can apply the following **before** your camouflage:

★ medication for your skin condition
★ sun protection
★ moisturisers (emollients)

You can apply decorative make-up **over** your camouflage.

For more help and advice please contact your BASC-trained camouflage consultant

NAME INSERTED HERE

on

CONTACT DETAILS INSERTED HERE

Your agreed skin camouflage products

Camouflage
brand

colour code

quantity

Camouflage
brand

colour code

quantity

Powder
brand

colour code

quantity

These are available:

on NHS prescription

on order at chemists

by mail order and online

More information

Although our consultants work independently of us, we are proud of the part they play in helping others to *face the world, with confidence*

SKIN CAMOUFLAGE CONSULTATION RECORD

PRIVATE & CONFIDENTIAL INFORMATION

NAME	
ADDRESS	
	Post Code

telephone – mobile	OK to ring?	YES / NO
telephone – work	OK to ring?	YES / NO
telephone – home	OK to ring?	YES / NO
e-mail		

contact medical team ? Yes / No	Doctor's name – Dept – Hospital address
	GP's name – address

letter required back to referring doctor ?	YES / NO	obtaining products on prescription ?	YES / NO

CONSULTATION DETAILS

DATE	TIME	VENUE

area to receive camouflage	
additional information, person's expectations	

	CAMOUFLAGE	SETTING POWDER
AGREED CAMOUFLAGE PRODUCTS	brand colour code	brand colour code
	COMPLEMENTARY	OTHER PRODUCTS
	brand colour code	brand colour code

sample & ingredients label sheet given? YES / NO	application & removal guidelines given? YES / NO	where to purchase products information given? YES / NO

follow up (date & result)
further consultation required :

CAMOUFLAGE PRACTITIONER'S NAME :

© basc\Tl\p-record   SIGNATURE .... date ....

14

Records should be stored in a lockable filing cabinet or secure files within your computer. When working with medical files, they will need to be returned to the appropriate ward or central filing system immediately after use. Documents from a legal firm must also be returned promptly to the sender. No copies should be made.

If you need to take photographic evidence of before and after camouflage application, you must obtain written consent from the person. You must state clearly why and in what circumstances the photographs will be used and they must sign to confirm their agreement. For example, you may intend the photographs to be used as evidence gathering for a portfolio for your private/qualification needs, for publicity within the workplace or to be used externally to promote skin camouflage. It is courteous to advise the person when their image is being used within the media and to also allow them the opportunity to object to any publicity.

working in hospitals and clinics
the frequency of the camouflage clinic will depend on each location's funding and people's needs. The camouflage clinic bridges all wards and is not confined to the obvious dermatology and reconstructive-plastic surgery departments. There is usually a process for in-patients to be directly referred to the camouflage clinic. However outpatients may require their doctor to request an appointment under the provision of the National Health Service in Great Britain. People would usually make their own arrangements with a private clinic.

There may be occasions when you are asked to visit someone to discuss the option of camouflage at a later stage in their care plan. Discussing camouflage (and when appropriate the use of postiche and prosthesis) can be a great morale booster, especially at a time when they really need support and reassurance.

working in a beauty salon or health spa
there is no reason why your camouflage service should be considered any different from other therapies provided. You may also provide supporting treatments which can be beneficial such as electrolysis, aromatherapy and so on. However, to avoid providing treatments which might conflict with any continuing medical procedures, it will be necessary for the person to discuss your therapy plan with their doctor and gain medical permission.

working in other settings
you may decide to provide your camouflage service as a home visit or in other settings. By making such visits you will be able to help someone who is physically or emotionally unable to travel to you. People can feel more relaxed in their own environment, or within a support centre or clinic specialising in their condition.

You may also wish to offer your camouflage service where those who have been victims of violence are offered counselling. Other specialised settings would include working within

- a high security hospital
- a prison
- an offenders' community programme
- an undertakers/funeral parlour
- a mortuary as part of the forensic pathology team

When offering your camouflage skills to such centres, it is vital that you can provide evidence of the specialist qualifications the centre may require, such as BIE (British Institute of Embalmers) or AAPT (Association of Anatomical Pathology Technicians) when working on the deceased.

It is vital you feel comfortable in the environment and that you make sure it is safe for you. Such precautions apply to practitioners working from their own home, or anywhere when working alone.

Because confidentiality must remain paramount, it may not be appropriate to visit people in your normal working uniform. You will therefore need to adjust your dress code appropriately and your camouflage kit can easily be transported in an ordinary bag. It is also worth mentioning that patients, especially children, will quickly recognise colour-coded uniforms and associate the colour worn with the degree of pain felt when that carer attended to their needs. To prevent psychological distress, particularly with children in a burns unit, it may be necessary to change the colour of your clothing worn during your camouflage clinic.

Wherever the consultation takes place, two vital environmental needs must be met: people's privacy must be guaranteed and you must work in appropriate lighting conditions.

correspondence with medical professionals

it is courteous and professional to reply to correspondence. Keep the information clear and concise so that it can be easily and quickly read. A medical practitioner will need to know the outcome of the consultation so that your recommendations are recorded on the patient's notes. This is especially important when the camouflage products are to be supplied in Great Britain through a National Health Service prescription. Itemise the products clearly in your letter and list the manufacturer's brand name, the identity colour name or code and the quantity required.

If an appointment is made but the person does not make contact, or does not attend, then you should first contact them. If the person declines the offer of your camouflage service, the referring medical practitioner should be informed because camouflage application may be a vital part of rehabilitation. If they, especially a Psychiatrist, believes the person to have been seen by you, and this is not the case, then further medical/psychiatric treatments may be affected.

medico-legal reports

the cost of camouflage products (including removal products and applicators) may be included in compensation claims after personal accident and injury. You may wish to become involved with this and offer your services to your local legal professionals. A legal protocol exists within Great Britain, and all those involved in personal injury claims must adhere to it. Following a normal camouflage consultation you would be required to complete a legal form or provide a written opinion. These would of course be confined to skin camouflage and not to medical matters. Most personal injury claims are settled out of court; however you are strongly advised to observe civil procedure rules and familiarise yourself with legal terminology. Rarely will you be required to attend court to reiterate or defend your opinion. Fees charged for consultation and medico-legal reports are costed within the litigation claim and you should take advice from the legal professional about your fee and when it will be paid.

insurance cover

an insurance policy is an essential safety net. At the time of going to press, BASC is unaware of any litigation made in relation to camouflage advice and application.

You should check that your employer has increased their insurance to include provision of skin camouflage. Most underwriters will include skin camouflage applications without increasing premiums. If you work under your employer's insurance umbrella, but also wish to provide a private service, you should obtain your own insurance. The Diploma awarded to graduates trained by the British Association of Skin Camouflage is accepted for indemnity purposes by medical and industrial organisations within Great Britain.

promoting your camouflage service

all advertising will depend on where the skin camouflage service is given. People who have lost confidence usually walk with their eyes looking downward; any advertisement should be placed at a level that will attract their attention. Keep the information clear and concise so that it can be easily and quickly read.

Seek permission before placing a poster with your local community's health and welfare providers. Do not make an appointment just to promote yourself - a well-drafted letter accompanying the poster, delivered by hand to the receptionist, is usually the most successful route. Also ask if a card can be pinned on the notice board, or that your details are kept on their database for future reference.

You may also wish to promote camouflage awareness by giving a demonstration and talk to community and support groups, or by contacting the relevant reporter on your local newspapers and radio.

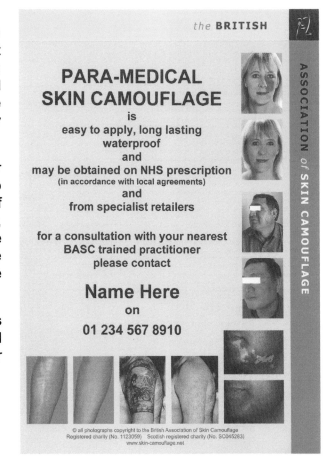

consultation fee

you may need to work out an appropriate fee for your service. This needs to be cost-effective and will depend on your expenditure. As a general guide, your fee should be similar to that of other services in your area, for example a consultation with a chiropodist or aromatherapist.

In some working areas it may be inappropriate or against policy to make any charge for your camouflage service. If the service is provided free, it may however be appropriate to have a charity collection box to allow people to make financial donations. Your workplace must give permission for a collection box. If permission is granted, but there is no earmarked charity, then a local skin support group or, indeed, the British Association of Skin Camouflage itself, may be an appropriate recipient.

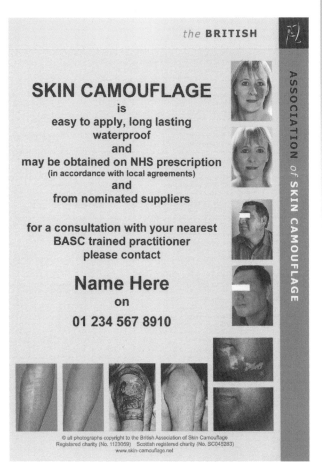

*establishing appropriate skin care routines
for use with camouflage products*

*there is a psychosocial implication that if our skin looks damaged or
uncared for, then other parts of us, or our character, may also be
flawed; but irrespective of how many products we buy,
or the effort we put into keeping our skin looking good,
our skin does not remain perfect – forever!*

establishing appropriate skin care routines for use with camouflage products

Constant marketing pressurises us to keep our skin looking flawless: it is no wonder that we will buy and try anything to improve it. This is often carried out with little or ill informed knowledge of both skin and cosmetic attributes. Although the outer layers of the corneum can be influenced cosmetically, over-stimulating the skin and applying inappropriate products is just as undesirable as neglecting it. Unfortunately we are often consumer led and can erroneously consider expensive products to be better for us than those that cost less. There is indeed a form of cosmetics snobbery when purchasing and it has to be acknowledged that marketing ploys entice us all to purchase products that may not really be essential. However, you should advocate the use of products containing UV protection, particularly for people with scar tissue and those with photosensitive skin conditions.

A suitable skin care routine should be encouraged where products used are designed to complement, or improve, the skin type and its condition. Not everyone will require the oft-promoted dogma of 'cleanse – tone – moisturise' or to exfoliate. Dry, dehydrated and mature skin and some dermatoses may not benefit from some skin toners or soaps, as they could remove too much oil from the skin. Equally the application of oil-based products to an oily skin may create a greater probability of blocking follicles.

Camouflage products are designed for use over sensitive skin and are generally termed as being minimal allergenic risk (within the EU), which means that all known sensitisers have been removed. However, all products, including skin camouflage, have the potential to irritate and trigger an allergic reaction. If someone experiences any erythema, itching, burning or unpleasant sensation, then the product must be removed immediately and the area cleansed (using alternative products) and a record made on the person's file. The person should be advised to seek a clinical patch test where the possible substances can be identified as causing the problem. The person must be given a sample of the suspected product together with labelling information for use at the patch test. This would include,

- age of product
- batch number
- brand name and product's colour code
- ingredient list
- manufacturer's name and address

Although a reaction usually presents within 15 minutes, it can sometimes take longer – up to three days – to develop. At the time of going to print, the British Association of Skin Camouflage is not aware of any confirmed allergic reactions to camouflage products.

regulations and legislation about the sale of products

until recently, manufacturers were under no obligation to disclose what is in their product. Obviously such information is essential knowledge to anyone with a clinically confirmed allergic reaction and to those who do not want to unwittingly place on their skin an ingredient that is offensive to them for religious and cultural reasons. A bonus is that the consumer can now appraise ingredients versus price when making a 'like for like' purchase. Manufacturers of camouflage products available in GB comply strictly with regulations laid down by the EU, USA and other countries concerning the safety of the ingredients, colouring agents and preservatives.

Ingredients are listed with the greater quantity first and then on a sliding scale to those <1% of the product. Such trace elements can be listed in any order. Any ingredient within the formulation that may affect the skin has to be listed separately under the heading of 'active ingredients' for products made for the USA. At the time of going to print, active ingredients do not need naming in cosmetic products sold elsewhere. However, that may change and most reputable companies will identify both active and non-active ingredients, even when they are not required to do so. Products sold to, but manufactured outside the EU, must comply with EU legislation. Camouflage products, toiletries, make-up, skin crèmes (including sunscreens) would generally be classified as "decorative cosmetics" within the EU. The USA has a different method of classification; for example moisturisers containing a sunscreen would be categorised as cosmetic drugs, those without sunscreen as decorative cosmetics.

Recent studies suggest that skin is permeable to nanoparticles that could filter through the skin and be swept up by the capillary and lymphatic system, which, in turn, may affect vital organs. Further research into the differences between corneum absorption and dermal permeability is being undertaken as well as any potential detrimental effects that frequent and prolonged usage may cause. Any product found to contain ingredients that can filter through the skin, or may actually alter the structure of the skin, will be reclassified as being a medication in the EU (some may possibly be referred to as 'cosmeceutical') and should, as such, only be available from pharmacy counters. Products that are innocuous will remain as direct over-the-counter sales. Camouflage products do not contain medicinal properties to alter the structure of the skin although most do contain sunscreen.

At the time of going to print the EU regulations have yet to include a shelf life date for products that remain unopened; manufacturers need only advise customers of a 'use by' date when the product has a shelf life of under 30 months. On products that could last longer (but can deteriorate after opening) the EU has amended existing legislation to include a 'period after opening' (PAO) symbol.

Not all toiletries, camouflage and decorative cosmetics require a PAO (especially those that are hermetically sealed) but those that do will have different timeframes – each manufacturer determines the life expectancy of a specific product. For example, lotions applied to the skin, such as sun protection crème should typically have a 12 to 18 month PAO but a shorter PAO is required for products designated for the eye or lip area. The cosmetics industry insists that most products can be used safely for longer periods – the PAO is meant to indicate only the time in which the product might be less safe, effective or pleasant to use. Products manufactured for sale outside the EU may come under different shelf life legislation.

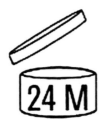

the number denotes the months, once opened, that the product should be used before discarding

However, no product will last indefinitely and will also rely on the consumer's hygienic practices, which means keeping the product contamination-free. As a general rule, when stored and handled correctly, camouflage products have a shelf life of 30 to 36 months or a PAO of 12 to 24 months. You must ensure that a product is safe for use. No one should rely solely on a date stamp : any product that looks different to how it should, emits an incorrect smell, feels wrong when touched or if you suspect it has been contaminated, must be thrown away. If the product has made contact with skin, then the area must be thoroughly cleansed.

keeping skin clean and hydrated

camouflage products are water-resilient and people will need to know which products are best used to remove the camouflage and for cleansing their skin. They will also need to appreciate what might unwittingly remove or lift their camouflage during wear.

Environmental dust and dirt, skin cells that have not desquamated, bacteria and waste products deposited from the evaporation of sweat all happily attach to the surface of the corneum, as will camouflage products, decorative cosmetics and any other topically applied product. To keep skin healthy it needs to be cleansed of those waste materials. Because the surface of the skin is waterproof it requires a cleanser that can remove dirt and also debris attached to the surface sebum. To do that we need to use a surfactant (wetting agent) such as soap (detergent) or an emollient (an emulsion of water, wax, grease or oils) as a soap substitute.

water, by itself, is insufficient to thoroughly clean the skin – the sebum, being hydrophobic, will repel it – we are naturally "waterproof". Usually when water is placed on the skin, it evaporates (using natural body heat to help do so). Prolonged immersion in water, such as swimming, will not affect skin camouflage. However, damp or wet camouflaged areas must be naturally air dried (not by heated hand-drier) or gently patted dry, not rubbed with a towel.

The skin, when warmed, can create a self-cleansing action that automatically 'flushes out' sweat pores by increasing perspiration. This action occurs in humidity, when in a sauna and when the skin is under an increased heat source. The normal function of perspiration will continue underneath the camouflage. Excessive perspiration and humidity can make camouflage products less stable on the skin, but will not remove them. The person may need to reapply their camouflage more frequently than others do.

Using *soap and water* together removes surface dirt well, but this method of cleansing can leave the skin feeling taut and dry (a sensation that has quite erroneously been associated with cleanliness!) and we usually apply an emollient (moisturiser) to counteract that. Sebum can be removed by frequently using detergents, soaps or an alkali which defat the upper corneum layers. This can lead to increased epidermal water loss, skin cracking and irritation. The good news is that healthy skin can regenerate the sebum quickly. Normal everyday use of soaps does not pose a threat, although for people with eczema or dry skin soaps may exacerbate the dryness. Scars are prone to dehydration when cleansed with soap and water. To avoid irritation, people must ensure that the soap is thoroughly removed from their skin.

Soap and water will quickly remove camouflage products from the skin – a point to remember when camouflage is applied to areas that are frequently cleansed, such as hands. Care must also be taken not to use toiletries that contain surfactants, such as shower gels or household cleansing products close to or over camouflaged areas.

A more gentle method of cleansing the skin is to use an emollient as a *soap substitute*. Emollients which have a higher percentage of water than oil are known as oil-in-water, while those containing more oil than water are known as water-in-oil emulsions. Cleansing milks and lotions are excellent to use for removing non-set camouflage products, especially during the skin camouflage colour matching process.

cleansing milks or lotions are generalised as being oil-in-water emulsions. Although those on sale are more complex than this, as a base principle a cleansing lotion usually contains a small quantity of detergent (and as such is excellent on oily skins) whereas cleansing milks do not (and are better for dry skins). Checking the ingredients list will confirm the emollient properties and if there is any soap in the formulation. Some brands are designed for use on dry, oily or normal skin, or for babies, or suggested for use on face, hands, etc. Emulsions containing antiseptic, antifungal and antibacterial active ingredients (such as tea tree) may prove beneficial to cleanse acne and rosacea skin. All emulsions remove camouflage products, but it may take more than one application to achieve that unless using a formulation specifically designed for that purpose. These products are used in conjunction with disposable cosmetic pads or facial tissues.

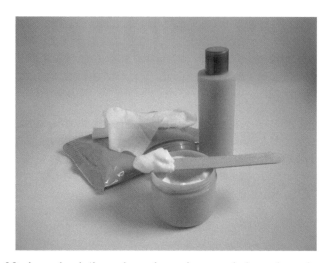

03 cleansing lotion, cleansing crème and cleansing wipes

cleansing crème and oils are generalised as being water-in-oil formulations. These may prove to be the answer for dry, dehydrated and mature skin (and for use over scar tissue), but may be detrimental when used on oily or acne skin. The oil in the formula softens the surface sebum (along with any attached debris) and is wiped off the skin with disposable cosmetic pads or facial tissues. With little effort, they are very effective at removing set camouflage products. Some cleansing crèmes contain a small amount of detergent, which can cause irritation when left in contact with the skin. If the skin feels too greasy after such cleansing, a gentle skin toner should then be used to remove the excess oil.

cleansing wipes are disposable cloths impregnated with soap substitutes designed to keep hands and skin clean and/or to remove decorative cosmetics. They work on the same principle but have the advantage of being a fully portable 'all-in-one' product, which frees the person from carrying several items or needing to use a sink. Cleansing wipes remove camouflage products and they are also ideal for the camouflage practitioner to keep their hands clean during the skin match process. Caution: brands may contain fragrance, soap and chemicals (designed to keep the wipes moist in their container) which might be a skin irritant.

exfoliants

some cleansers incorporate mild exfoliants. These dissolve or scour the corneum, which in turn will remove flaking dry skin and help reduce outbreaks of comedones. They may also slightly improve the appearance of fine wrinkles by removing the upper layers of the corneum; however there is concern that excessive use could increase photosensitivity and lessen the skin's natural defence mechanism. Exfoliators must be thoroughly cleansed off as prolonged contact may cause skin damage. By their very nature, exfoliants will remove any topically applied product along with the squames.

Exfoliating agents frequently used in cleansing toiletries are bran, oatmeal, AHAs and BHAs (Alpha and Beta hydroxy acids). These acids are derived from food, plants and vitamins, the most common being lactic (milk), citric and tartaric (fruits), salicylic (willow), glycolic (sugar) and retinoic (vitamin A). AHAs and BHAs are known photosensitisers and the use of sun protection must be strongly recommended to everyone.

Over the counter facial masks and peels are purpose exfoliants for infrequent use at home. Salon strength range from superficial (gentle) topical treatments to the slightly deeper micro-dermabrasion peels using specialist equipment. The use of concentrated exfoliants and LASER resurfacing/surgical dermabrasion for scar reduction and cosmetic purposes are procedures that should only be offered by qualified medical professionals.

Always follow the manufacturer's instructions and comply with professional aftercare advice when using exfoliants.

toning products

skin toners (including skin tonics and astringents) are designed to remove oiliness, but they will not prevent the skin from producing oil. They are also promoted as products which 'tighten pores' and give a cooling refreshed feeling to the skin. However, anything applied which is colder than the skin will automatically trigger the skin's natural mechanism to tighten pores (reducing the secretions of sebum and perspiration) and to contract the superficial blood vessels – all of which give an invigorating sensation until the skin reverts to its natural state. Splashing the skin with cold water has the same effect.

Toners fall into two groups. Generally those for oily skins usually contain astringents such as witch hazel together with solvents and alcohol. Care should be taken to use an alcohol-free product when working with communities who forbid its use due to religious and cultural constraints. Those made for dry skins contain little, or no alcohol plus a humectant such as glycerine. Both forms usually contain plant extracts to soothe the skin and give a pleasant smell but have little long-term therapeutic effects to the skin. Plant extracts, such as lavender, contain substances that can trigger a reaction (allergen) and may increase photosensitivity. Alcohol and some plant extracts will dehydrate the skin.

Toners are not essential products and should be used with caution on those with dry, mature or sensitive skins and scars as they could intensify dehydration. A gentle skin toner may be useful to remove any excess oil left on the skin and to remove soap residue. Gently wipe toner over the skin using a disposable soft cosmetic pad.

emollients (moisturisers)

cosmetic and toiletry manufacturers provide the public with a variety of products with the sole aim to moisturise, nourish and soothe specific areas of the skin. Some contain vitamins, sun protection factors, bronzing colours, bleaching agents and chemicals which are designed to help the skin retain its natural moisture (or slowly release hydrators) - some will even suggest that they will remove wrinkles and rejuvenate the skin. Dermatologists agree that the inclusion of sun protection is very important but are continuing to question how efficacious other ingredients, such as vitamins, may be when applied topically.

Moisturising products (and soap substitutes) are based on the oldest skin crème formulation known. The Greek physician Galen (circa 130–201) made a crude emollient by mixing water into a blend of molten beeswax and olive oil. Unfortunately it was little thought of until the 19th century when Mr Pond (using liquid paraffin instead of olive oil) reinvented the "cold crème". It was nicknamed cold crème because, when applied, the water content evaporated quickly thus cooling the skin. A note of caution, white soft paraffin contained in ointments, emollients, etc., may rot the rubber seal of your washing machine!

Today's moisturisers are very sophisticated products but still work on the principle of leaving a fine film of oil (wax or grease) over the corneum. That helps prevent natural evaporation with the trapped water automatically hydrating the skin. It has to be argued that if you cleanse your skin with a 'cold crème' then you have little need for a moisturiser! The most effective moisturiser would be a product such as petroleum jelly, olive oil or lard! Indeed Anita Roddick (founder of The Body Shop) commented as such at the Cheltenham Literature Festival (2002) when she remarked that Tahitian ladies use animal fat to keep their skin feeling as soft as velvet.

Moisturisers can be applied with clean fingertips or by wiping the area with a disposable cosmetic pad containing the product. When applying a moisturiser you need to allow time for the upper layers of the corneum to absorb it (the maximum timeframe is 20 minutes) and then wipe off the residue. Moisturisers should not be applied directly before applying camouflage or decorative cosmetics, unless the manufacturer suggests otherwise, as they will make the camouflage or cosmetic less stable on the skin. You can also disperse emollients into bath water by placing some on your hands under a running tap. Although this form of bath can be beneficial to skin, it will dislodge any applied camouflage.

An emollient or bland oil can also be used to massage scar tissue.

scar massage

you should advise people of the importance of finger massage to scar tissue. The short time taken at a consultation to explain why and to describe the method is amply repaid by the results. In some cases people may have already been advised, but it is worth clarifying.

Many professionals believe that improvement cannot be expected from massaging a scar that is more than five years old. However, massaging scars sustained many years previously has shown to be of noticeable benefit. Massage will certainly not harm and is always worth trying, but the older the scar the longer it will take to show any improvement. It is good if patients can improve the condition of the scar, which may reduce their need to continue using camouflage products.

People are strongly advised to seek their medical advisor's agreement before starting massage therapy, which should begin as soon as possible after the scar has been sustained. After surgery, this means once the sutures have been removed and the scar is "healed and sealed" to withstand enough force to move the skin over the underlying structures.

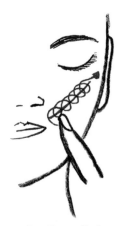

People should use a lubricant and move their fingertips in a tight circular motion over the scar, giving special attention to raised edges and places where hardness can be felt. Ideally this exercise should be carried out daily and continued for a minimum of one year. It is worth noting that even when the scar is less visible, massage is beneficial because it keeps the scar tissue supple and the surface hydrated.

Should camouflage application be required immediately after massage, then any excess greasiness will need to be removed by blotting with a tissue. Do not massage over camouflaged skin as the friction and/or oil will remove it.

using fingertip in a tight circular motion, massage over the scar

As well as massage, hypertrophic and keloid scar tissue may benefit from silicone sheets and gel dressings.

silicone dressings

it is not known exactly why the application of silicone can flatten, soften and fade scar tissue, but research indicates that when successful the improvement remains permanent. Silicone works best on new scars, particularly hypertrophic and keloid, although improvement has been shown when used on very old scar tissue. Some keloid and hypertrophic scars may not respond at all and sadly silicone has little effect on atrophic scarring.

silicone sheeting is marketed in various forms – some are self-adhesive and others require a backing sheet to adhere it to the area. Silicone sheeting can be cut to size to fit exactly over the area concerned. Some products are thinner than others are, but all are light and easy to wear. Some can be washed clean and reapplied, giving several applications, whereas others may need to be renewed daily. Camouflage is difficult to apply over silicone sheeting and, being proud to the skin, its margin will be noticeable. However, the sheeting can be worn during the night with the person applying camouflage over their scarring during the day.

silicone gel gives a very fine transparent layer and will be easier to manage over digits and joints. Because only a thin layer is required it becomes almost undetectable. The gel is easily removed by cleansing the skin.   Camouflage and decorative cosmetics can be applied over the set silicone, which is a bonus as the scar is then less visible. If camouflage is not being used, any glossy effect of the gel can be minimised with the application of cosmetic powder to match the surrounding skin tone.

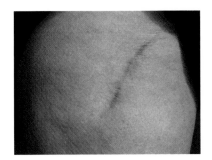

*03 erythematous scar
(following hip replacement)*

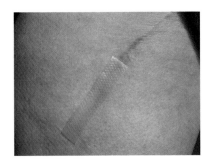

*03 some silicone sheeting is
not suitable for skin camouflage
to be applied over the top*

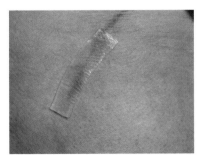

*03 but can be worn, as
manufacturer's instructions
(without the skin camouflage)*

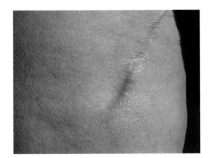

03 silicone gel covering half of the scar

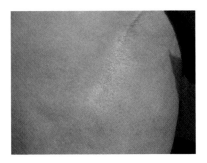

*03 with skin camouflage applied over
the silicone gel (to half the scar)*

sun protection

given that there is no such thing as a 'healthy tan' constantly keeping out of the sun may not always be easily achieved. It is essential therefore to protect skin from the harmful rays of the sun, which can be equally damaging on a cloudy day and during winter months. Sunbeds and sunlamps are just as damaging as natural UV.

Manufacturers recommend that sun protection is applied half an hour before going out. It cannot be over stressed how important it is to reapply the product frequently to maintain protection. Products available may protect the skin from UVA and/or UVB. It is advisable that the ingredient list is checked to see that <u>both</u> UVA and UVB rays are being screened. Camouflage products usually contain titanium dioxide (which is a natural and excellent UV reflector) which helps to screen skin from UVA and UVB and some have a registered SPF value.

understanding the sun protection factor (SPF)

the manufacturer must substantiate all SPF values. SPF values are calculated by taking the time an average skin can tolerate exposure to UVB before erythema, then multiplying that timescale by the sunscreen properties of the product. If a person can tolerate unprotected UV exposure for five minutes before erythema, and purchases a product with an SPFx30, then 5 x 30 = 150 minutes (2½ hours), which is the maximum total exposure time before the product should be reapplied. As a guideline, dermatologists suggest a minimum SPF 30 for all skin groups and reapplication at intervals more frequent than personal maximum exposure time.

People who are classified as being skin groups 1 to 3 need greater protection than those in groups 4 to 6 - but there remains the potential for all skin groups to burn when exposed to intense sun, especially when the person is more used to living in a country with less sunshine.

Camouflage products alone will not provide sufficient protection from the sun. To give additional protection, sunscreen should be applied before and under camouflage application. Sun protection products not containing oils can be carefully applied at regular intervals over the camouflage.

ideally the best suntan comes out of a bottle!

For those wishing to have a sun-tanned skin, it is best to achieve the colour by artificially staining the skin, (see page 99).

3

*camouflage products, tools of the trade
and professional working practices*

*tools can unwittingly create psychological barriers
– there is much to be gained from a "hands on approach"*

camouflage products, tools of the trade and professional working practices

With a growing awareness of the need for products to camouflage successfully, manufacturers have produced ranges of specifically designed crèmes and powders. These differ from decorative cosmetics because they have greater covering qualities, are highly pigmented and, when applied correctly, are resistant to water and smudging. However, no product should be considered totally rub-proof and the and people need to be made aware that there may be minor transfer and soiling to clothes and bed linen.

All brands have accompanying literature explaining how to apply and store their products.

Manufacturers suggest their products have a stability-durability time on the skin of between 8 and 24 hours. The timescale will obviously vary according to their lifestyle, skin condition and daily hygienic practices. Some brands may require an emollient to be applied before (and under) the camouflage – others may recommend that a gentle skin toner is used first to make sure the area is totally free of any natural sebum or residue from a skin cleanser.

Throughout this book we do not mention any particular brand name or colour code. This is a deliberate policy because all manufacturers will inevitably increase or decrease their product range over time. It is important for you to update your product knowledge regularly and ensure that your working kit includes only those products that are currently available. Another reason, and something that will influence your decision-making, is that locally and internationally some brands are more readily available than others are. As you would expect there is a broad price range, but most products cost no more and are usually less than decorative cosmetics. It is worth remembering that a little camouflage will cover a large area of skin and that there should be little need to reapply it for several hours during wear.

At the time of going to print there are several brand names within GB currently listed in the Drug Tariff and the Monthly Index of Medical Specialities (MIMS) Borderline Substances – that is circulated to the medical profession and pharmacies. This means that the products have been scrutinised by the Advisory Committee on Borderline Substances (ACBS) at the Department of Health for reimbursement on Form FP10 (which is a general practitioner's prescription). Camouflage may also be prescribed in hospitals when the product is on the hospital's formulary. However, Borderline Substances are at the doctor's discretion and it may be that some practitioners will refuse to write a National Health Service prescription for camouflage crèmes and setting powders. Likewise there is no guarantee that any listed product will remain in *MIMS* indefinitely or that other brands will pass the National Institute for Health & Clinical Excellence (NICE) scrutiny and be added to the list. The brands of camouflage listed will also be available from direct sales without prescription, however some brands may not be obtainable internationally and you will need to consult the manufacturer for individual country availability.

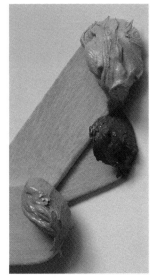

03 ratio 1 part dark mixed with 2 parts pale = acceptable coloured camouflage crème

There is a vast choice of pre-mixed skin tones and complementary colours that are used to conceal hyperpigmentation (and tattoos) before the skin match is applied. Where there is no exact skin matching shade, or suitable complementary colour, you will need to mix colours together in varying quantities. Due to costs and time involved we do not recommend mixing more than two colours together to achieve an acceptable skin match. Although not necessarily endorsed by any manufacturer, one brand of camouflage can be used in conjunction with another (or mixed together) with excellent results.

There is also an ever-increasing range of camouflage products available as over the counter sales from chemists, supermarkets, cosmetic retailers and from the Internet. It would be impractical to work with every product on sale, as the choices would overwhelm you and the person seeking your advice. But do familiarise yourself with as many of the products as you can. Start by getting as many samples as possible: this will help to prevent overstocking and buying colours that you will not use. Manufacturers provide printed shade cards and, while these might not be ideal (because printing distorts colours slightly) they will at least give you an indication of their colour range.

When you have got your samples you can compare the differences among the brands for texture, durability and stability. The viscosity of the crème can differ noticeably among brands: some will flow on easily; others may be more difficult to spread. The siting of the camouflage will also affect durability: in areas where friction may occur, the camouflage will be less durable than to areas where the possibility of any 'rubbing off' is eliminated. Climate and people's workplace and lifestyle must also be considered as these can affect stability of their camouflage. Those who live in a cold climate, or work in a cool environment, will find the camouflage more durable than those who live or work in hotter and more humid conditions.

The camouflage selection process will inevitably be dictated by your personal preferences, but always take the following important patient-related questions into account:

- what brand will best suit their needs and lifestyle?
- what are the cost implications?
- where will they obtain their supplies?

camouflage products available

cosmetic concealers
are good for masking hyperpigmentation under the eyes and mild erythema. Colour corrective concealers and powders are also available, which follow the complementary colour theory (see page 53 – does green cancel red?). Concealers are usually applied before the application of cosmetic foundations; colour corrective powders are applied over

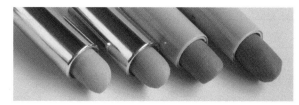

03 skin coloured cosmetic concealers

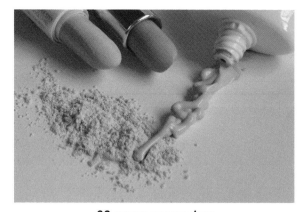

03 green concealers

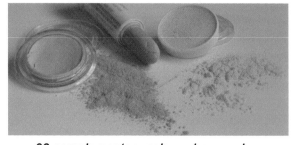

03 complementary coloured concealers

specialised foundations

are very useful for covering leg veins as they have a greater covering power and stability than decorative cosmetics as well as some degree of water-resistance. Unfortunately these products may not give sufficient durability or covering for many dermatoses or a tattoo. Available from theatrical make-up retailers are dry palette colours, which are activated by adding water or medical alcohol before application to the skin by sponge or brush. These products give exceptional staying power although the alcohol can dehydrate the skin and irritate sensitive skin – especially with prolonged and frequent use

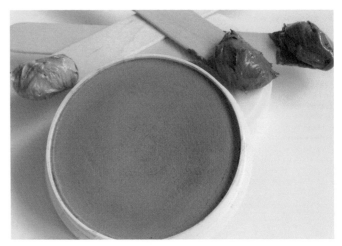

03 theatrical crème and pancake make-up

camouflage crèmes

are best described as highly pigmented crèmes that require setting with loose powder. The pigment is designed to mimic skin colour and, where necessary, to create features such as false freckles, beard shadow and veining – complementary colours are also available

Leg and body camouflage crème is more liquid and easier to apply to those areas

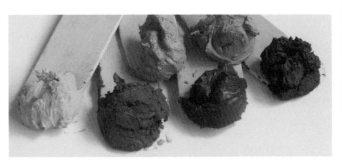

03 camouflage crèmes

Crèmes are waterproof once correctly set, which allows the wearer to take full part in social activities, including swimming and water sports, to bath and shower, and have protection against inclement weather giving confidence in the stability of the product. Most manufacturers recommend that it may take several minutes before the camouflage is fully set and waterproof – and this should be explained to people. However, blotting the camouflaged area with a damp cosmetic sponge, (see page 83) can accelerate setting time. When first applied camouflage appears to sit on top of the skin but does look more natural after a short time. This is because the camouflage will mix with the skin's natural sebum and, to an extent, sink into the upper layers of the corneum. Indeed it could be argued that camouflage crèmes help to keep skin hydrated by forming a barrier that is oil based.

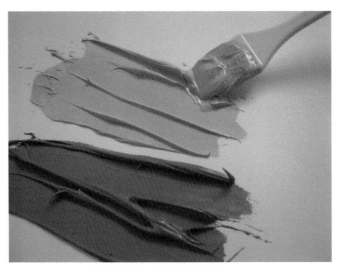

03 leg & body camouflage crème camouflage

loose setting powder

is needed to set camouflage crème, which helps fix the product to the skin and enhance waterproofing properties. Colourless is ideal as it will not alter the colour of the camouflage crème. Some loose powders are designed to mimic skin tones, which can increase or modify the camouflage colour underneath. People, for personal reasons, may prefer to use unperfumed used as powder. Talc and powders will give a matt finish to the camouflage. Cosmetic bronzing and shimmer powders are useful over set camouflage to give lustre.

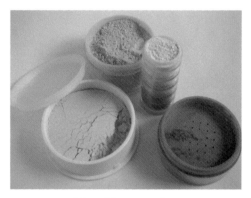

03 setting powders

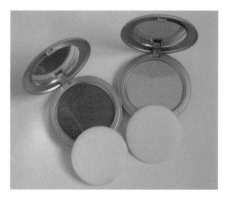

03 compact powders

Should the powder dull the skin or give a ghostly effect, the solution is to use one that does not contain titanium dioxide, or a product based on rice powder.

Compacts are also available with a dual compartment for crème and powder. These can be useful to carry round in a pocket or bag. Powder camouflage and duel compacts are available from specialist make-up retailers.

powder camouflage

for people who do not wish to use oil-based formulations, there are highly pigmented camouflage powders (micronised minerals) that adhere to skin primed with an emollient. These powders, available as loose and in compact form, can be used to good effect on conditions such as acne and rosacea. Although they might have less covering properties and durability, most will be water resilient.   For maximum cover they can be used as the setting powder over crème camouflage.   Problems, as previously mentioned, will occur with powders containing titanium dioxide

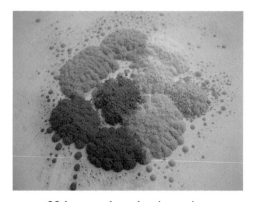

03 loose micronised powders

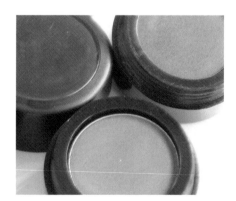

03 micronised powder in compact form

This form of camouflage does not require setting powder and there is no need to blot with a damp sponge cloth.

fixing spray

with an aerosol or pump action, is designed to go over camouflage (set crème and mineral powder) and give greater durability to areas where the camouflage may be rubbed off, for example under cuffs, necklines and bra straps. Fixing spray can also be used to seal a complementary colour before the skin match is applied.

Fixing spray is colourless - a light mist gives a semi-matt finish and subsequent applications will build up to a full gloss effect - which is a very important outcome for many camouflage applications where the surrounding skin has a natural glow. Fixing spray is also available in a matt finish.

airbrush foundations

airbrushing is a method of applying highly pigmented fluid cosmetics via compressed air and a spray gun. Normal camouflage products are too thick to pass through the mechanics of airbrushing so a special fluid foundation is required. The foundations contain the co-polymers that give the product its long-lasting and water-resilient properties. There is no need to set the airbrush foundations with powder or blotting. There are 'dewy' finishes available if the result seems too matt or fixing spray can be applied. The foundation can be disturbed on the skin and removed from the skin by the same criteria as normal camouflage products.

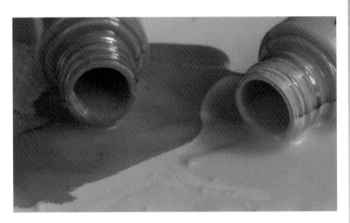

03 airbrush foundations

Airbrushing is also used for creating faux tan by spraying the tanning product onto the skin.

skin plastic

is designed to fill in atrophic scarring. However, it remains questionable whether these plastics are sufficiently stable to take into account movement involved in daily life as they retain their soft consistency and are easily dented. Embarrassment would result from the product falling out and, in addition, skin plastics are difficult to cover with camouflage. It is not recommended that skin plastics are glued into place or any form of adhesive strip applied over the plastic to secure it to the skin. Depending on circumstances, the person could be issued with a prosthetic to plug the atrophy. Their medical practitioner may consider injecting a filler.

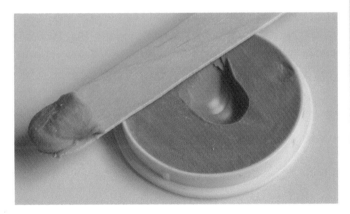

03 skin plastic

However skin plastic and silicone fillers can be put to good affect when working on post mortem skin.

products designed to stain the skin

obviously a product that is designed to colour the skin for several days has immediate advantages over traditional camouflage. Always use sparingly as a little goes a long way. The colour should be confirmed as acceptable before the stain is applied to the whole area: alcohol wipes can be used to remove test areas.

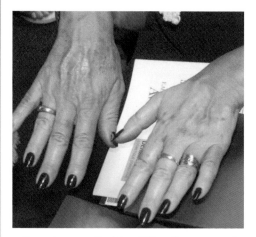

faux tan applied to vitiligo fingers and right hand – left hand for comparison

© *Alida DePase BASC Member 2158*

faux tan

some products contain a guide colour – which does not indicate the finished tan. Always consult the manufacturer's instructions as application techniques may vary, and comply with their recommended safety or protective clothing, especially when using an airbrush.

Faux tans work best on depigmented skin such as vitiligo; unfortunately, they usually darken any hyperpigmentation and are ineffective over moderate to severe erythema.

Thankfully these products are now less likely to streak or appear amber-orange on the skin. Although the current range of colours is best suited for skin groups 1 to 3, manufacturers are working on darker stains. Some products include a Sun Protection Faction (SPF), but none can be considered as a substitute for applying sunscreen protection. Products containing a guideline colour make application easier. Most products take up to 24 hours to develop the colour fully. The colour fades as the skin naturally desquamates; most faux tans will last 3 to 5 days before reapplication is required.

Skin groups 4 to 6 may require subsequent applications, every eight hours, to build up the colour, but at the time of going to print a faux tan to mimic their natural colour has yet to be manufactured. However, faux tan products – whether crème, mousse, liquid or airbrushed – can be very useful even when the skin match is not exact. The faux tan will diminish the contrasting skin colours when applied under camouflage to areas where there is less durability, such as hands. For patient evidence into the efficacy of using faux tans. please see Products Available To Camouflage Hands – Vitiligo page 143

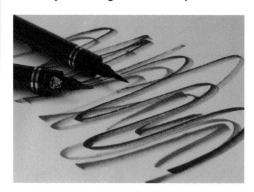

03 lip stains

lip stains

can have greater durability than camouflage crèmes or long-lasting cosmetic lipsticks. These are used to create a lip shape, or to infil lips where the natural colour has changed or is missing. Those available in tube and pen formats are ideal for people who would be embarrassed to use a product that looks identical to a decorative lipstick. Staining pens have disposable felt tip applicators which ensures hygienic practices

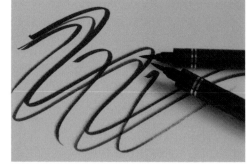

staining pens to create eyebrows and to outline eyes

may prove to be the better choice for the person whose eyes have a tendency to water. The pens are water/smudge proof and can be used to great effect when eye lash and brow hair is missing.

03 stains to use as eyeliner or for brow hairs

tools of the trade

during the camouflage skin matching process you will need skin cleanser, cosmetic tissues or pads to remove mistakes and a mirror for people to view outcomes. You will need to confirm when working in some specialist areas, such as secure units, that they allow the use of mirrors and applicators. You also need to appreciate that an application tool creates a barrier between you and people – whereas using fingertips and a 'hands-on' approach reassures the person that they are not 'untouchable'. Someone who has been the victim of violence may also back away from a brush, spatula or similar object because they will perceive it as a weapon coming towards them.

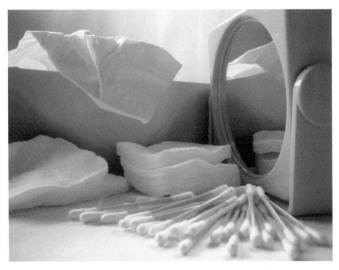

03 tissues, cotton pads, cotton buds and mirror

You must comply with your workplace Health & Safety Code of Practice and due to strengthening infection control, hospitals now encourage the use of disposable items. It may be that you will need to show the person what applicator(s) they need to purchase (and suggested retailers) but then use disposable equipment during the consultation. A nice gesture is to offer them the ones used on their skin to use at home rather than throwing them away.

You may need some type of spatula to remove cleansing crèmes from their containers. You can use wooden spatulas, which once used are then discarded, or metal or plastic spatulas that can be re-used after being cleaned aseptically.

However, it is more economical to use wooden cocktail sticks when selecting camouflage colours to create a skin match. You could use wooden orange sticks, but this can prove expensive as you will use so many of them. Plastic orange sticks, which can be cleaned and re-used, are another option, as are slender spatulas, but you will invariably pick up too much product from its container – using a cocktail stick will prevent that.

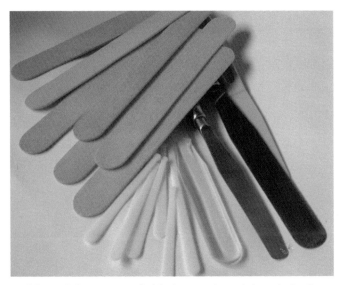

03 spatulas are available in wood, metal and plastic

It would be inappropriate to use a spatula, stick or any form of palette, for testing the skin colour match (or to transfer the product) directly against the person's skin.

brushes

the best brushes on the market are not necessarily the most expensive. The brush hair must be soft (to avoid any discomfort) while being sufficiently firm to maintain precise control. A brush is ideal for small areas, narrow scars, creating lip line and infil, eyebrows and when working close to hair and lash lines

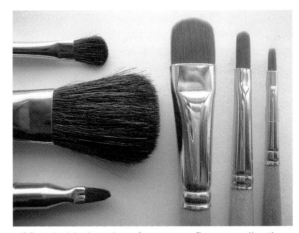

03 suitable brushes for camouflage application

disposable brushes

eliminates the need of aseptic cleaning between use. Disposable sponge-tipped applicators can be used, as long as they are soft and have a very fine edge. A brush, disposable foam-tipped applicator or a cotton bud is a good tool to use when creating 'fake faults', such as moles and veins (see page 87)

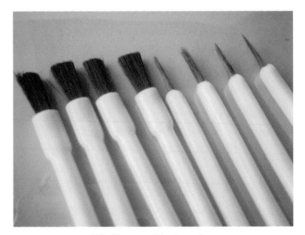

03 disposable brushes

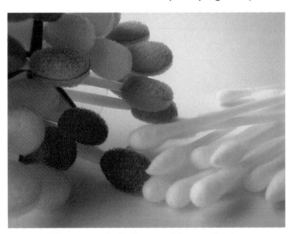

*03 suggested disposable applicators
to recreate faked faults*

A **powder** or **blusher brush** is essential to brush off excess powder and to brush vellus hair in its natural direction of growth. Males may prefer to use a dry, soft-hair shaving brush instead. A large soft brush can be used to apply powder camouflage. However it is not an appropriate tool for applying setting powder because you will not pick up a sufficient amount of the product

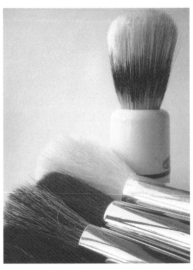

*03 selection of brushes suitable
for brushing off excess powder*

sponges

there are environmental concerns that restrict the sale of natural (sea) sponges and because latex is a known sensitiser, any sponge used must be made of synthetic materials. Sponges, which are used by beauty therapists and make-up artists for treatments such as facemasks, are inappropriate, as are bath sponges.

Sponges are excellent when a very delicate touch is needed, such as for rosacea or to cover bruising.

Cosmetic round sponges, including those that need to be used damp, give equal results. All will create a fine layer and are the easiest to use when the skin colour is needed to show through the camouflage to give a very natural effect. A soft dry sponge can be used to apply powder camouflage.

The fine edge of a ***cosmetic wedge*** can sweep under lower eyelash lines, around nostrils and be very useful for feathering camouflage, especially into the hairline. A wedge is ideal for applying fixier spray to the face.

Being inexpensive sponges are considered disposable applicators.

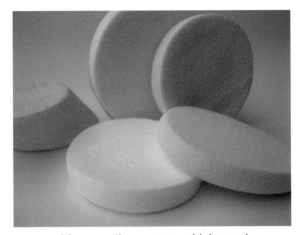

03 cosmetic sponges which need dampening before use

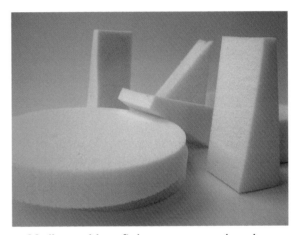

03 disposable soft dry sponges and wedges

stipple sponges

are essential for breaking up a solid colour, creating multiple freckles or recreating beard shadow. Synthetic sea sponges can also be used to create random mottling. They do not need to be dampened before use. You must aseptically clean and dry them thoroughly before re-use.

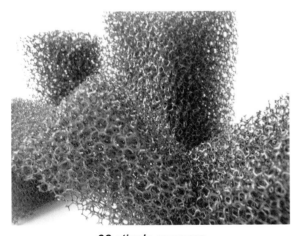

03 stipple sponges

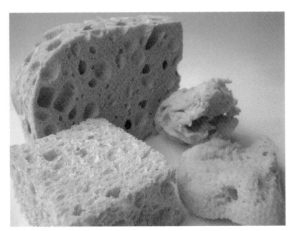

03 synthetic sea and cosmetic sponges for stippling

sponge cloths

are used for blotting the powdered camouflaged area to hasten setting and to remove any excess powder. These cloths are used damp and should always be used to blot over skin that has hair stubble. The used cloth must be clean for each person. If you use dry or damp cotton wool over hair stubble you may unwittingly achieve a 'Father Christmas beard' effect, embarrass them and spend time carefully picking off the fluff from their stubble! The same principle applies to using cotton wool pads instead of powder puffs.

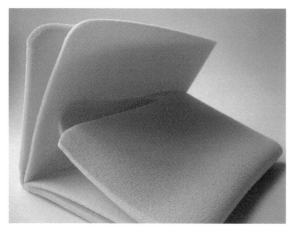

03 soft sponge flannel used to blot larger areas of camouflage

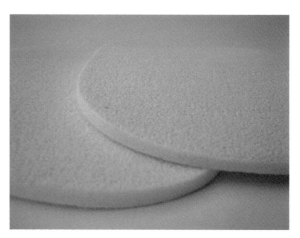

03 soft sponge cloths used to blot smaller areas of camouflage

powder puff

the best type has velour on both sides and ribbon handle; this form of puff can also be used should you have the need to protect the person's skin from the side of your finger or hand.

Use one puff per person. However, if you are running a hectic clinic you can cover the puff with soft gauze, which can be discarded after each use. The gauze helps to keep the puff clean and free of possible cross-contamination. Using a cosmetic tissue to protect the puff is not recommended as the powder tends to slide off the tissue and not transfer well onto skin. After cleaning as described below, make sure the velour is patted in its correct direction before drying

An alternative is to use large synthetic, fibre-free cotton wool pads, which make reasonably good disposable powder puffs when wrapped in gauze. Natural cotton wool is not recommended for applying powder, even with muslin wrapped round it. This is because it can cause allergic reactions and the fluff can stick to the skin.

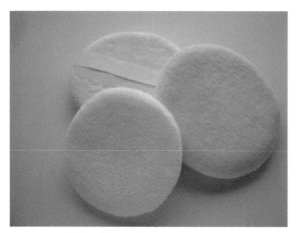

03 double sided velour powder puff with ribbon handle

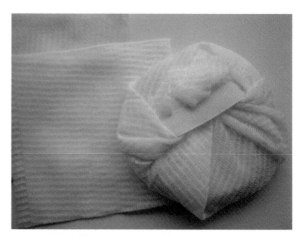

03 puff wrapped in disposable gauze

airbrush

makeup artists have used this method for many years within the film and television industries and this concept has now come onto the high street. The industrial heavy duty (and weighty) and expensive compressors are impractical for home use. Airbrushing kits now filtering into retailers have smaller sized and cheaper priced compressors for salon use and portable kits which are battery operated or use compressed air canisters as the propellant (instead of a compressor). There are also handbag-sized atomisers and aerosols available. However, people might find it difficult to transport the equipment to enable them to adjust their camouflage during wear. People would also need to check before travelling by air that the equipment (especially compressed air canisters) is allowed in their luggage.

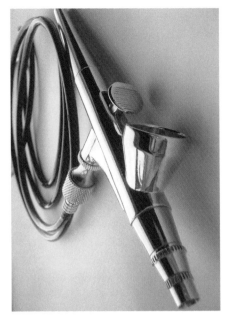

03 airbrush nozzle

**for psychological and hygienic reasons you will discover that
the best tools of the trade for everyone is to use
your palm as a mixing palette and fingertips to apply crème camouflage**

guidelines for cleaning tools

if your applicator equipment is for use on more than one person, then all items must be cleaned with antibacterial soap to remove all traces of the camouflage product, then thoroughly rinsed before being aseptically cleaned and dried before reuse.

You must comply with the Code of Practice within your place of work. Keeping your equipment in an aseptic condition means using an appropriate solution, such as those used by make-up artists and hairdressers. However, some solutions can rust the metal caps on brushes and turn sponges yellow, so it is best to experiment on old tools first to see what effects different solutions might have.

You may need to rinse applicators under clean running water to remove any strong chemical odours and traces of the cleansing solution that could trigger an allergic reaction. All cleaned applicators must be totally dried before storing away.

People also need to be advised on how to clean applicators used and how to handle and store their camouflage products.

storage

you will need to store equipment and products in a hygienic condition and safe place. Camouflage products, cleansers, toners and emollients should be stored away from direct sunlight. Ideal containers are plastic boxes with airtight lids which are easy to keep aseptically clean. It may be necessary to store products in a refrigerator when your environment is equatorial, however you will need to bring products to comfortable room temperature before use.

You may prefer to decant products into smaller containers which will save you from carrying heavy or large loads, or if there is a need to create an isolated range of products as a safety precaution against potential cross-infection. Containers and equipment used for decanting must be aseptically clean to eliminate any cross-contamination. All transferred products must be clearly labelled with the manufacturer's name and product identity code or name, batch number, the recommended use-before date and the date you transferred the product.

Unfortunately, in Great Britain not all brands are immediately available as over the counter sales and usually have to be ordered through a pharmacy or through specialist suppliers. Because people may experience some delay in obtaining their camouflage, it is sensible to keep enough sample stock so that you can give them a small amount following their consultation. This will allow the person to perfect their application skills and practise any adjustments needed before their ordered supply arrives. To comply with current legislation you must also give them a list of the product's ingredients and manufacturer's contact details.

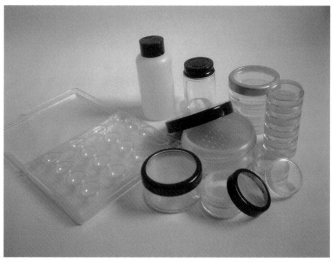

03 selection of suitable empty containers

professional working practices

you must comply with the health, safety and hygiene codes of practice laid down by your place of work. There should be no occasion for you to wear a mask or similar barrier clothing when using camouflage products, unless the workplace specifically requires you to do so. Hair must be secured in a way that it will not fall either onto people or into products. Jewellery, especially to wrists and raised rings on fingers, should not be worn as they could scratch people or harbour germs. For the same reason, fingernails must be kept short and clean. It is recommended that you do not wear false nails or any form of nail varnish as these can be allergy sensitisers.

Your hands need to be kept clean. A tub of wet-wipes is ideal for this and avoids you interrupting the consultation with frequent visits to the sink. Your palm and finger can be kept clean by using wet-wipes and this will save your brushes and sponges being used during the skin match selection process.

The work area must obviously be kept clean and tidy at all times. Disposable wet-wipes can be used to clean the area and couch paper to mop up any spillage. Couch roll makes good disposable surface protectors, and can also be used to protect clothes.

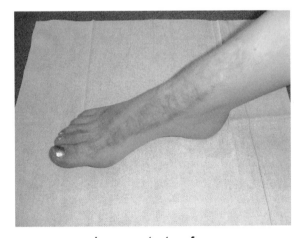

always protect surfaces
© The Camouflage Club at the Burned
Children's Club : BASC Member No. 2163

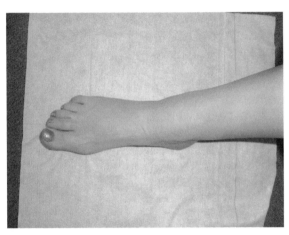

burn scar with camouflage applied
© The Camouflage Club at the Burned Children's
Club : BASC Member No. 2163

You will need to protect people's clothes from camouflage products, but don't embarrass them by insisting that clothing should be removed when rolling up a sleeve or trouser leg allows dignity. Disposable cosmetic capes are useful for protecting clothing, but do not offer any 'modesty' protection if made of clear plastic. Ask people to clip back their hair only if it will interfere with the camouflage application.

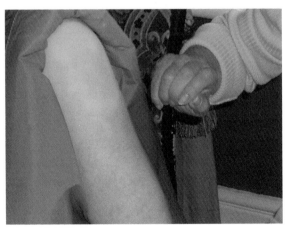

clothing protected by a cosmetic cape
© BASC

People need to be in a comfortable position. A chair is the usual choice, although a couch might be needed when applying camouflage to the person's trunk or legs. A couch is not recommended when applying facial camouflage because the face muscles droop slightly in repose – it is better if people sit upright. Sit beside the person and do not use a table, couch or trolley as a barrier between you.

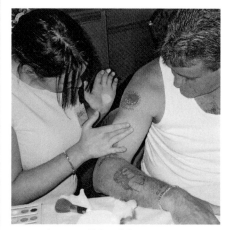

always sit beside someone
© BASC

Never use a magnifying glass to view the person's skin and never hand them a magnifying mirror, as these will exaggerate their dermatosis and also make a successful camouflage application unconvincing. However, people need to see what you are doing, as well as hearing how and why. When you are working on an area of skin that is not in their comfortable line of vision, they need a hand-held mirror. Always suggest to the person that they view the application with the mirror at arm's length (preferably the end result via a wall mirror), as that will give a true indication of how others will see their camouflage.

For some reason camouflage on the lower leg (from knee to ankle) can look good to anyone seeing it from the front, but to the person looking from a standing position at their legs it can appear as a bad skin match or too powdered. People need to look at their legs in a wall mirror to counteract this optical illusion.

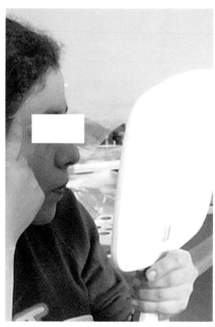

there is a risk that the person will hold a mirror too close to their face (model kindly posed especially for this photograph)
© BASC Member 2160 (at Aniquem, Peru)

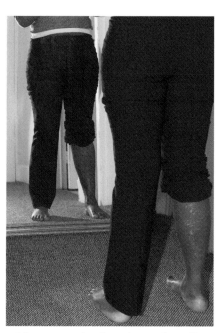

02 person viewing via a mirror the camouflage applied to her lower legs

You need to be able to work without stooping and in a position that gives you easy access to the workstation. Always sit people in in optimum lighting conditions, next to you and, most importantly, involve them in making decisions about their preferred method of application and the skin match colour selection.

*light - sight – pigment
appreciation of the colours
in camouflage products and skin*

*the judge in the Gilbert and Sullivan operetta Trial By Jury boasts
that he quickly climbed the ladder of success by marrying a rich
attorney's daughter who was elderly and not very pretty but
could "pass for forty-three, in the dusk with the light behind her"
– indeed, such lighting is the ideal to flatter,
but useless for camouflage skin match consultations!*

light - sight - pigment
appreciation of the colours in camouflage products and skin

Your main objective during the camouflage consultation with the person seeking your advice is to create an acceptable skin match to their natural skin colour. To do that efficiently and quickly you need to appreciate your lighting-working environment and understand the colours within the camouflage products (and how to mix colours to achieve the right outcome) and the pigmentation to the person's scar or dermatosis and its surrounding skin colour will make product selection easier.

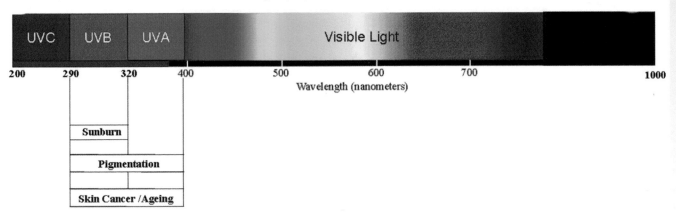

spectrum : wavelength indication range of light visible to the human eye
© Lynton Lasers

light

Isaac Newton did not just consider why apples fall to the ground – he also played a major role in analysing the composition of visible (white) light. By using a glass prism, Newton demonstrated that light can be split into the colours of the rainbow and that the dispersal sequence remains constant (circa 1660). He is also attributed as being the first to turn this visible spectrum of light into a circle of colour. LASERs emit monochromatic light, which means that they discharge just one colour (or one fixed wavelength) that travels in a straight narrow beam, whereas IPL emits a range of colours, or wavelengths, between 560 and 1200 nanometers, which is known as broadband light. Both target specific structures in the skin, such as capillaries, melanocytes in skin and hair, and pigmented lesions. The light, which will create heat, is predominantly absorbed by the target which will then destruct with minimal damage to the surrounding skin.

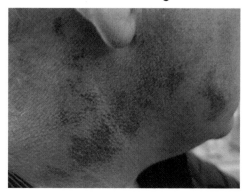

naevus flammeus
© BASC Member 2019

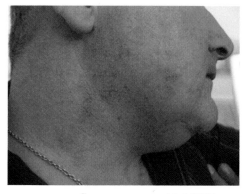

naevus flammeus : post LASER
© BASC Member 2019

When applying camouflage to create a skin match it is essential to work in good lighting conditions, which is daylight or natural (white) light. To appreciate why daylight is best, you need a basic understanding of artificial lighting and the colour interaction this can have on people's skin and the camouflage products. One of the most flattering lights is a gold-rose (sunset) colour as it warms the colour of the skin and gives it a healthy glow. Hairdressing and beauty salons, make-up counters in department stores and clothing shops will often use this form of lighting to make customers feel good and, hopefully, encourage them to spend more! However, when the product is viewed under other forms of lighting, its colour may not be so flattering or may totally change. The result is that the product may be put to one side, forgotten and unused.

Tungsten (incandescent lamp) lighting gives a warm glow, produced by using the orange-red end of the spectrum. It creates healthy looking skin, but can intensify erythema and any yellow tones to the skin. It will also give a false yellowing to camouflage products when creating the skin match.

Although manufacturers have done much to improve fluorescent lighting, it can cast a blue-green colour over the skin, making someone look tired and grey. Camouflage products will appear greyish during the skin match process. Low energy light bulbs may also have the same effect.

When working in an area where there is no direct light, or where the lighting conditions are less than adequate, use a portable desk lamp with a 'natural' light bulb. These recreate normal (sun)light and are available from craft shops and some specialist hardware stores.

Obviously it is better to work under natural daylight, but if you are next to a window that could be overlooked, it should either have opaque glass, blinds or a net curtain to shield people from observation. When under direct sunlight someone with photosensitivity should be advised to apply their sunscreen before the consultation. Ideally, if your camouflage station is next to a window, the glass should have a UV filtering system fitted to help protect people.

As long as the camouflage skin matching process has been achieved in good lighting conditions it will not matter if people apply their camouflage under tungsten or fluorescent lighting conditions at home. When camouflage looks good in natural light, it will remain true under artificial lighting too. Unfortunately, if the initial skin match is achieved under artificial light, it may not be good under natural or other forms of lighting.

sight

each human eye has between 6.3 and 6.8 million cones and 110 and 125 million rod-shaped photo-receptors within the retina which, together with nerve fibres, form part of the mechanism of sight and transmit that signal to the brain. The cones detect colour – there are three types red, green and blue. Colour blindness occurs as a result of the absence or malfunction of one or more of these three. The rods provide the distinction of light and shade, which gives form (or shape) and perspective to our vision.

In simple explanation, the human eye 'sees a colour' when the corresponding beam within white light is reflected back from the viewed object to the eye (all other light rays are absorbed). For example, the eye recognises that grass is green (in daylight or by artificial white light) because the grass absorbs all the other rays and bounces the green light wave back to the eye. When the natural light source is removed, the grass is seen as dark grey or black (and at night by (yellow) street lighting, the colour of grass is seen as dark brown).

Anything seen as white is reflecting back the whole 'rainbow' to the eye and something black is absorbing all the wavelengths. This is the reason why white minerals, such as titanium dioxide, work as a natural sunscreen by reflecting the sun's rays off the skin.

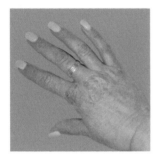

01 psoriasis

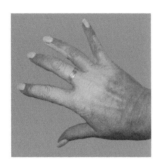

01 "flash back white" when a photograph is taken with flash activated

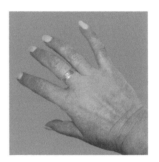

01 minimised when taken without the flash activated

Titanium dioxide, zinc oxide and calcium carbonate are used to give degrees of opaqueness to the camouflage crème or powder. Consequently, the eye does not see, for example, erythema either because of the opaque quality of the camouflage formulation (the light bouncing back the whiteness into the eye) and/or because of the 'browning' effect created by overlaying the area with its complementary colour. Unfortunately that principle also applies when a photographic image (with the flash activated) is taken of camouflage products and decorative cosmetics which contain those light-reflecting minerals; the camouflage will appear whiter than the surrounding skin. Ways to minimise this unwanted "flash back white" are discussed in page 101.

It goes without saying that you must possess good colour vision – a requirement for make-up artists and other professionals whose work involves using colour. However, no two people have identical colour vision and unfortunately, with age, our ability to see colour diminishes.

It is vital to acknowledge that people will see their skin colour and the suggested camouflage slightly differently to you. If either you or the person wear tinted or photochromic lenses to corrective spectacles, then the glass tint may also affect the colour of the skin and camouflage products viewed. It is essential that people are involved in selecting a skin colour match; a consultation resulting in a camouflage practitioner insisting that their choice overrides that of the person seeking your advice can only be regarded as a failure. People will inevitably will not use the recommended colour/s as they will regard them as unsuitable.

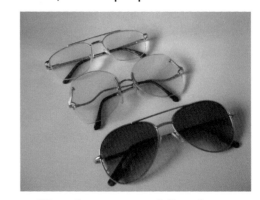

03 make sure prescription glasses do not affect colours viewed

pigment

in 1766 Moses Harris published the first organised colour wheel which was based on Le Blon's (a German theorist) earlier discovery (c.1731) that a comprehensive range of colours could be obtained by using just the primaries. The colour cone is a method that represents analysing colour in a logical way. It may be easier to appreciate the colour cone by thinking of it as planet Earth. The colours known as the primary, secondary and tertiary hues are placed at the equator.

Primary hues cannot be created by intermixing with any other colour, hence their name, but when mixed together they create black. They are:

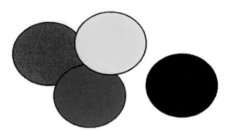

- red
- yellow
- blue

Secondary hues are created when two adjacent primary hues are mixed:

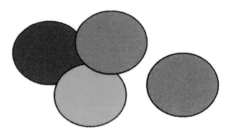

- orange   (red mixed with yellow)
- green   (yellow mixed with blue)
- purple   (blue mixed with red)

we create brown by mixing two adjacent secondary hues together

Tertiary colours are the primary and secondary colours mixed in ratio parts as they progress from one colour to the next.

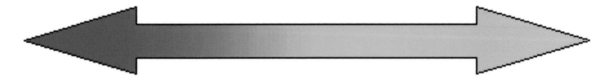

When describing the tertiary colours, the smaller quantity used to modify the main colour always appears first. For example:

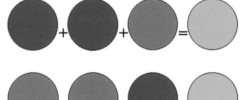

- a mix containing more blue than green achieves a greeny-blue colour (which we usually call turquoise)
- a mix containing more green than blue achieves a bluey-green colour (which we usually refer to as jade)

A similar mixing process is used to create other colours, for example the colour named as flame red (red modified with orange) or lime green (green modified with yellow).

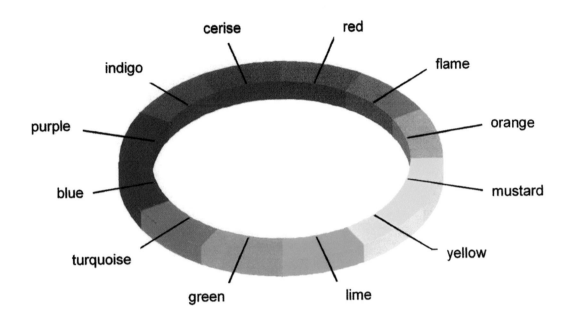

primary, secondary and tertiary ring

Having created an equator containing the primary, secondary and tertiary hues, the colour cone can now be extended by the addition of white or black. In this example, pure white is placed at the North Pole and the South Pole is given pure black. In this way, travelling along the axis from white to black, through the centre of the earth, there is a line of various degrees of grey.

The outer surface of the earth can now be modified with white or black. Hues coming away from the equator in an upward sweep will have a proportion of white added; the closer to the pole, the whiter the hue becomes. Colours modified by white are usually called tints, but may be called pastels or highlights.

Hues coming away from the equator in a downward sweep will have varying degrees of black added. The closer to the pole, the blacker the hue becomes. Colours modified with black are usually called shadows, but may be called shades or lowlights.

Colours known as tonal now need to be allocated to complete the colour cone. Tonal colours are concerned with adding grey when the colour travels at a right angle from the outer surface towards the central axis. Whether it is a dark or light grey depends on which 'hemisphere' of the cone the colour is in. The closer to the axis, the greyer the colour becomes.

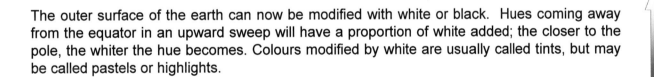

The colour cone, now complete, can be cut vertically to reveal 'slices' of colour – each one would show a snapshot of its place round the equator, plus all modifications by adding white, black or grey.

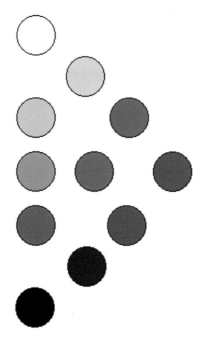

We usually refer to pigments by name rather than refer to their place in the colour cone. However, this does require us to form a colour-name association that is totally reliant on having experienced the colour before, for example canary (yellow), robin (red), raven (black). Cosmetics manufacturers also like to give their colour mixtures fancy names, which may perplex the purchaser until the item is seen! For example, 'Nectar Shimmer' – is this a yellow-gold or an iridescent dark honey colour?

Manufacturers of camouflage products name their colours or use numerical coding, the latter, unfortunately, giving the purchaser no indication whatsoever of the product's colour and some names being equally confusing until the colour is viewed.

does green cancel out red?

the complementary colour wheel theory is based on mixing together two opposite colours from the 'equator' ring to create a grey-brown colour. For example, red is exactly opposite green - theoretically, by applying a fine layer of green over red, the red is cancelled out and the eye receives a mixed (grey-brown) colour message.

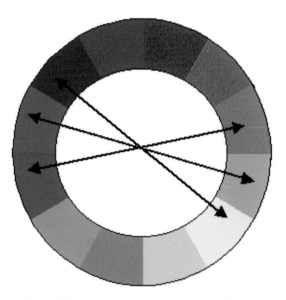

ring with complementary colours indicated

It follows that applying a complementary green should cancel out a ("ruddy") vascular complexion and erythema, but you will frequently find that the skin then takes on a ghostly appearance, or that you now have green skin to camouflage!

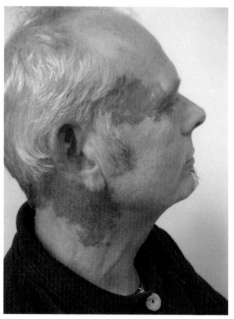

port wine stain
(colour analysis being blue-red)
© BASC

53

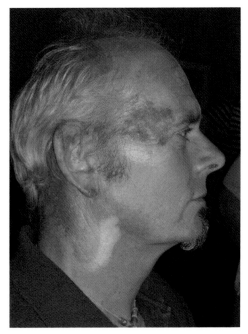

with green coloured concealer applied

© BASC

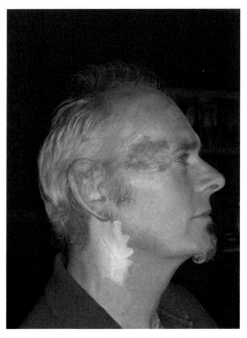

with green coloured camouflage applied

© BASC

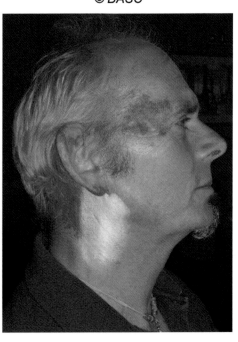

with white camouflage applied

© BASC

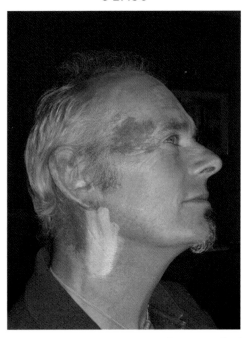

with cream coloured camouflage applied

© BASC

You will also discover that using white or cream colours as the complementary will create a similar problem to adding green – you now have white or cream coloured skin to camouflage….

Before applying any complementary colour you must analyse the colour of the area requiring camouflage because vascular dermatoses, bruises and erythematous scars are not pure hues, neither is any skin group and very rarely are tattoo inks!

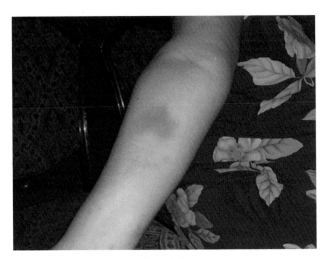
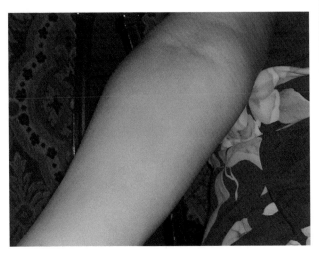

03 bruising   *03 bruising with camouflage applied*

For camouflage, the complementary colour theory needs to be expanded. Using the example of vascular conditions, you will discover that it is not 'just red' – it is usually modified with blue from the capillaries, taking the erythema within the blue-red or purple-red section of the complementary colour ring. The correct complementary colour will therefore depend on the ratio of how blue-red or purple-red the erythema is. The same principle applies when analysing the colour of any dermatosis, scarring or tattoo.

The complementary to blue is orange and purple is yellow. You will discover that 'purple-blue' erythema will need an orange with a hint of yellow, and (rather than apply a lime-green complementary) 'purple-red' erythema will be easier to block out using a yellow modified with a hint of orange. Either will require the addition of white or a cream colour to bring the complementary colour to a pastel for skin groups 1 to 3 with less added for skin groups 4 to 6.

why do we see "blue" when blood is red?

this is an optical illusion, blue has a shorter wave length and travels through the skin quicker than any other colour.

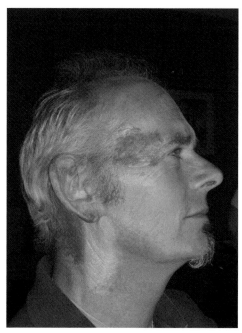

*with mustard coloured
camouflage applied
© BASC*

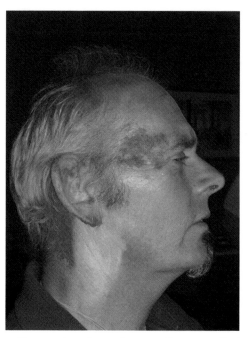

*with peach coloured camouflage applied
© BASC*

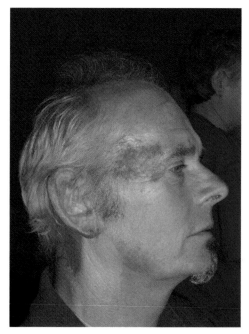

*with skin match coloured
camouflage applied
© BASC*

However, you must always first consider whether one (or two layers) of the skin match is sufficient without the need to apply a complementary underneath. In the illustrations you can see that **no** complementary was required – one layer of skin match was sufficient!

Experience will show you that conditions usually requiring a complementary colour are brown lesions (such as melasma, which usually have a blue undertone) and tattoos.

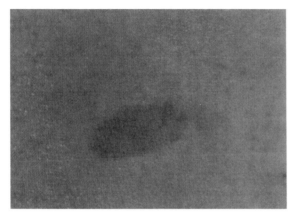

café au lait
© BASC

feint blue shadow appears, which a complementary would rectify
© BASC

analysing the colour to a tattoo
a tattoo is either monocolour (totally black) or polycoloured and outlined with black.

monocolour tattoos
although the complementary colour of black is white, 'black' is rarely pure and usually has an undertone of blue or green. Blue-black is usually prominent in new tattoos with green-black becoming evident as the tattoo ages and with exposure to UV light. When applying white as the complementary, you will discover that a tracery of the tattoo shows through the white. This is because the blue or green within the black has not been totally cancelled out. By analysing the composition of the black, you will be able to create the correct complementary by adding orange (for blue) or red (for green) to the white.

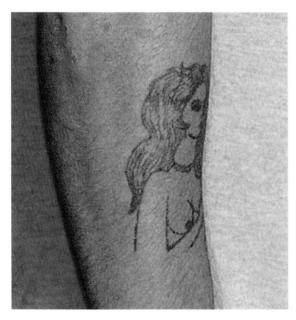

01 monocoloured tattoo

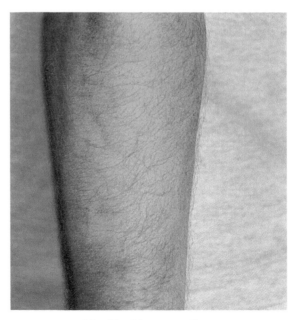

01 with skin camouflage

polycolour tattoos

when confronted with a polycoloured tattoo it would be an impracticable task to create a complementary to cancel out each colour and the black outline; and it would be too time consuming for the person to reproduce the tattoo in its complementary camouflage colours. The simple solution is to study the whole area and analyse the overall colour composition of the tattoo and then create the complementary colour that will block it out.

When considering a tattoo that has an overall blue-green colouring, it will be cancelled out by applying complementary orange-red. If it is predominantly blue-purple, then the complementary will be orange-yellow. The complementary will need to be adjusted by degrees from pastel for skin group 1 to full hue for skin group 6 (see page 109 for skin groups).

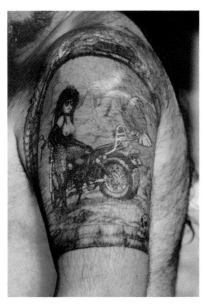

01 polycoloured tattoo

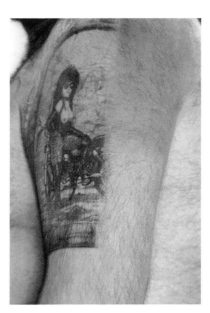

01 tinted orange is the complementary for this predominantly blue-green-black tattoo, with skin match camouflage applied to cover half the complementary

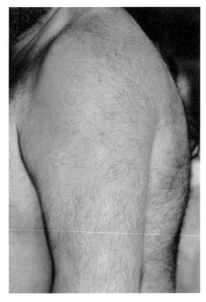

01 with skin match camouflage applied over the complementary

If the tattoo is predominantly yellow-orange-red in colour, to avoid any problems associated with the application of green, it may not be necessary to apply a complementary at all. The simplest method may be to apply two or three layers of skin matching camouflage. However if a tracery remains you will need to mask the black outlines using the appropriate complementary.

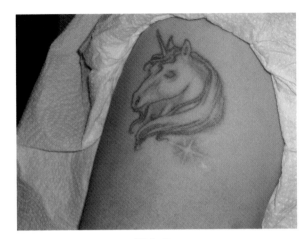

03 tattoo

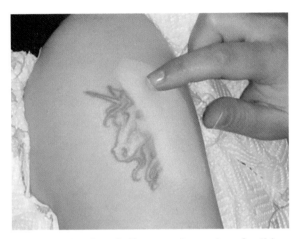

03 tinted yellow is the complementary for this predominantly purple-black tattoo

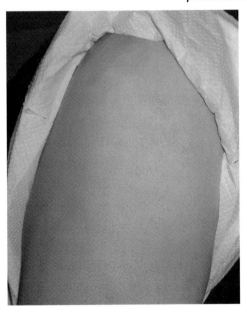

03 with skin match applied over the complementary

Manufacturers produce pre-mixed camouflage complementary coloured crèmes, as well as white and cream, from which you can mix and modify any colour.

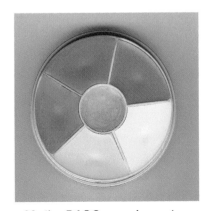

03 the BASC complementary colour wheel

colours in skin

for an efficient skin matching camouflage consultation, all the above now needs to be put together with our appreciation of the person's skin colour and their skin condition requiring camouflage.

The overall colour of dermatoses and scars can be broadly classified as being:

- hypopigmented; where the skin has less pigment than its normal colour

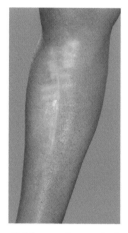

01 hypopigmented

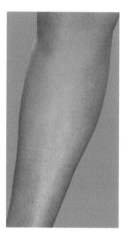

01 after skin camouflage

- hyperpigmented; where the skin has more pigment than its normal colour

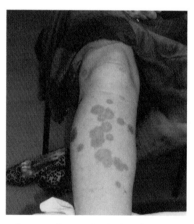

hyperpigmented skin lesions
© BASC Member 1022

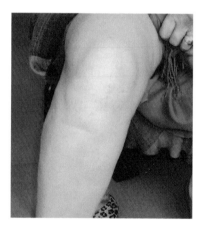

after skin camouflage
(without complementary to mask "blue")
© BASC Member 1022

- erythematous: where the skin is redder than normal

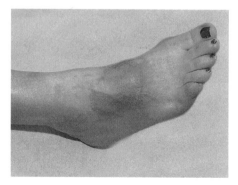

02 erythematous skin lesion

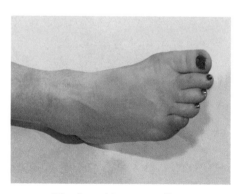

02 after skin camouflage

changes to skin colour

everyone's skin will be pale in areas where clothing has shielded it from direct sunlight; we all have slightly darker skin on the outside of our arms and backs of our hands. When the area to be camouflaged crosses from the light to the darker areas of skin (such as in the forearm) colour choice is simplified if the darker area is matched first and a little white (or cream colour) is added for the pale inner arm. Also consider people who work outside or who are going on holiday when the original colour match could prove incorrect. People will need an additional colour to modify their skin matched camouflage to the changes in their skin when exposed to UV. If you are uncertain how the skin may, or may not, tan – then ask them. People will need the corresponding red-yellow-brown to add to their camouflage to mimic the changes made by the sun, or an independent darker camouflage colour. It may be necessary to see them in winter and again in the summer for corrective skin matching. The same principle applies to people whose skin will change colour due to on-going medical treatment such as chemotherapy.

natural colours in skin

the predominant (base) skin colour is a visible mixture of the melanin (brown), subcutaneous fat (yellow) and capillaries (blue-red). It is the base tone that you aim to match acceptably with skin camouflage. However, do not be distracted from the base tone by any undertone (natural fault) that shows through the skin. These, for example, can present as excessive blue-red (where capillaries are more visible) or yellow-brown (from freckles). Undertones, when required, are applied over the skin match to create true camouflage (see faking faults section)

Although someone's skin colour can be classified by their genetic make-up (country of origin) these parameters have become less defined in today's cosmopolitan society. The British Association of Skin Camouflage therefore feels it is inappropriate to suggest skin colours by race, religion or ethnic origin, refers to skin base colour grouped by how the skin reacts under UV as discussed in page 109.

Irrespective of ethnic origin, skin colour can be classified under two base tone groups – those that have blue-red and those that have yellow. You will discover that the majority of people are yellow toned and few people are categorised as being blue-red (the blue-red base tones are most frequently found in skin groups 1 and 6). When in doubt, there's a simple test you can use.

Always involve them and explain what you are doing and why (although, to avoid offence, you will need to modify the terminology used to describe the base skin tone as "cool" (for skin group 1 and 6) and warm (for skin groups 2 to 5)

Apply a small dot of rose-pink and mustard-yellow camouflage crème to the skin close to, but not on, the area requiring camouflage. Without intermixing them, spread each colour very gently over the skin. Whichever colour disappears, or appears less obvious, is the base skin tone.

Sometimes you may find that you have someone where the skin colour test does not work successfully – the person has equal yellow and blue-red tones – when it will make your camouflage choice exceptionally broad.

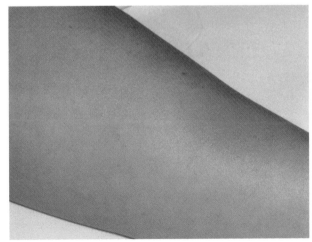

03 skin group 2 : where person has equal cool and warm undertones

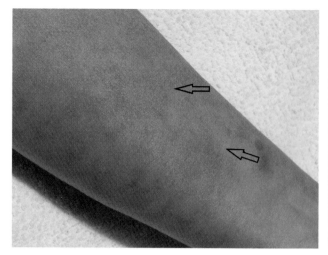

03 skin group 1 : the rose-pink is less obvious

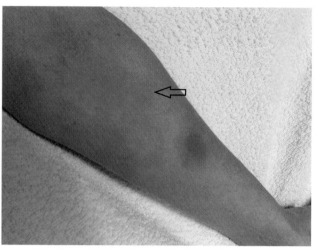

03 skin group 2 : the mustard-yellow is less obvious

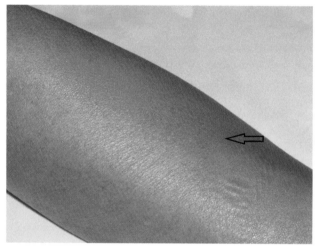

03 skin group 3 : the mustard-yellow is less obvious

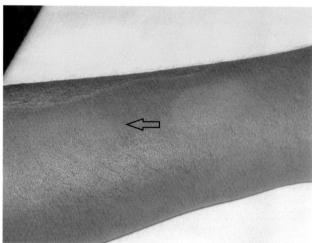

03 skin group 4 : the mustard-yellow is less obvious

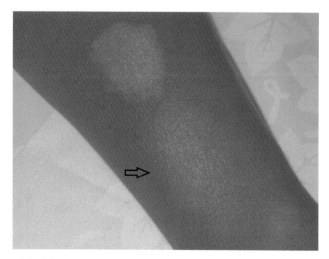

03 skin group 5 : the mustard-yellow is less obvious

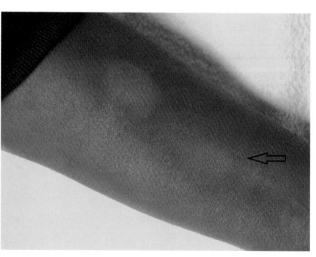

03 skin group 6 : the rose-pink is less obvious

colour in products

for successful camouflage, yellow-based skin requires a complementary and skin matching camouflage with yellow undertones; blue-red-based skin needs products with red undertones. To make selection of skin matching colours easier, you will need to appreciate whether the product has a red or yellow undertone.

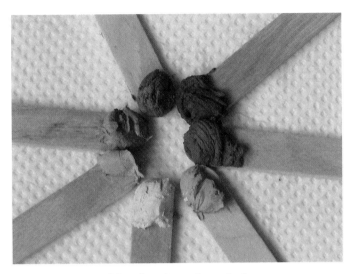

03 yellow based products

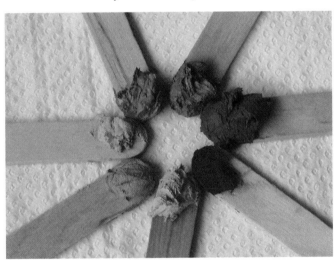

03 red based products

When the camouflage appears dull, even grey against the skin, it is because there is too much yellow in the product and the skin tone is blue-red based. You will have to reselect the colour or add pink to the skin tone mix. The same analysis applies to yellow base tone skin – the camouflage is too pink! This is an important principle to remember, especially when using complementary colours. If, for example, a yellow complementary is needed, but the person's skin is blue-red-based, then there can be an overall greying to the skin tone match. In this example, the complementary needs to be slightly more orange or even pink.

The skill of the camouflage practitioner is to quickly be able to:

- identify the base skin colour correctly
- identify any undertone to the skin correctly
- analyse the colour of the dermatosis, scar or tattoo to it's overall colour
- recognise which camouflage products are red or yellow based

*guidelines for a successful consultation
and camouflage application*

*with the exception of camouflaging a decorative tattoo,
the person should have gained medical permission for camouflage
to be applied, or have a prior medical diagnosis for their dermatosis*

guidelines for successful consultation and camouflage application

consultation

make sure both you and the person are comfortable and that you are working in correct lighting-privacy conditions; they will need to take away with them all the necessary information, including the brand/s and colour code/s of the acceptable camouflage used, and you will need to record that information on their file. People, with them taking charge of its safety, must remove any jewellery that could interfere with the camouflage application.

People can be very nervous when they come to see you and you will need to put them at their ease and dispel any anxieties they may have in using skin camouflage. You may need to assure them that skin camouflage is designed to give a normal colour to their skin and should **not** be confused with make-up or beautifying cosmetics. Allow the person to indicate their problem, do not assume what you can immediately see is what is causing them distress. Some people may need time to accept their new (camouflaged) image. In such cases, apply only a delicate layer of camouflage to give moderate cover. Over time, the person can adjust and gradually increase their camouflage to full density. However, some people only require the discolouration to be less obvious and do not want total coverage. Each person presents a new challenge – do not assume everyone requires an identical outcome!

At first people may feel that the routine might be too time-consuming, which is one of the reasons why you should keep your camouflage selection and application method as **simple** as possible. The person needs to feel confident that they can easily manage their camouflage routine - the more they practise, the more proficient they will become and the quicker their technique will be. Within a very short time they will become expert in their camouflage application.

For hygienic reasons we recommend camouflage is removed each day. This will also allow people to apply their skin medication (including silicone gel treatment for scarring), sun protection and moisturiser and encourage them to inspect their skin for any changes.

You must advise people not to continue with their skin camouflage if there is any change to their dermatosis, or their normal skin, until their medical adviser has given consent.

Some people may prefer to reapply camouflage immediately after removal, cleansing and inspecting their skin. There have been no reports at the time of going to print, that camouflage products, when immediately reapplied, cause harm or dermatological problems.

contraindications

a simple acronym to remember is **STOP** – do not apply camouflage over a skin that appears to be,

Suspicious

Transferable

Open

Purulent

Conditions generally contraindicated to camouflage application include,

- allergic reactions
- bites from fleas, mosquitoes, lice and mites
- blister, ulceration and pustular lesions
- bacterial infection, such as cellulitis, impetigo
- fungal infection, such as tinea (ringworm), pityriasis versicolor
- viral infection, such as herpes simplex (cold sore), herpes zoster (shingles), warts
- infestation, such as scabies
- illnesses that visually manifest on skin, such as chickenpox, measles
- occupational/contact dermatitis
- open wound
- skin cancer
- sutures
- undiagnosed rashes and some photodermatoses (such as actinic dermatitis)

preventing cross-contamination

if you are suspicious that any tool or product has become contaminated, then you will need to dispose of it immediately. All caps and lids should be replaced immediately on bottles, tubes and tubs, which will also prevent deterioration by oxidisation.

To avoid cross-contamination and maintain good hygiene,

- never put fingers or used application tools directly into any product
- never touch another person's skin with used applicators
- always empty sufficient powder onto a clean tissue and pick up the powder from there with the puff
- tap off any excess powder from its applicator – do not "blow away the excess" because the moisture from your breath will contaminate the remaining product and the applicator

Should there be a need to create some protection between the side of your hand and people's skin, a simple solution is to hold the powder puff by the ribbon in the crook of your finger. It would be inappropriate and uncomfortable to the person if you use a tissue or sheet of couch roll for this purpose.

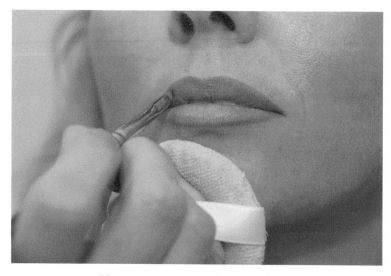

02 use a powder puff as a protector

If your workplace requires you to wear protective gloves, then it would be impractical to use the 'palm' and 'fingertip' application methods described. If this is the case, you will need to substitute the words 'palm' and 'fingertip' for appropriate tools. Unfortunately people will not receive the psychological benefits from a "hands on" approach. It may be that your risk assessment officer will revise the code of practice for skin camouflage application – which is, of course, topical, non-invasive and in full compliance with contraindications.

You need to advise people how to handle their skin camouflage products in a hygienic way and how best to remove camouflage products, cleansers and emollients from containers. If they use a sponge or brush to apply camouflage, then that too must be kept in a clean and hygienic condition, as will any powder puff or brush used. People must be advised always to wash their hands before starting to apply their camouflage, never to share their camouflage products or application tools with others and to discard any product when the shelf life expires and should they suspect it has become contaminated.

The skin and area close to that requiring camouflage must be clean of any dirt or cosmetics. However, only cleanse the skin if necessary (otherwise you will suggest to the person that they are unclean) and only remove decorative cosmetics on the affected area. If you ask them to remove their make-up you will not unwittingly embarrass yourself, or them, by removing decorative cosmetics to unaffected skin. Where appropriate, ask the person to bring their normal decorative make-up to apply over the finished camouflage.

Clean your hands directly before starting the camouflage application. If you clean your hands immediately after shaking hands with people you will unwittingly give the impression that they are 'unclean'.

creating an acceptable skin match
the first part of the consultation is for you to create an acceptable skin match. To do that you will need to,

- assess the area requiring camouflage, giving consideration to the depth of the discolouration and the surrounding skin colour to be matched
- assess the skin condition and lifestyle to ensure you use appropriate products
- assess and discuss which application method will be most suitable for them

Do emphasise to people that creating an acceptable skin match can take time – it is not always achievable at the first attempt. Do not be discouraged if it takes several attempts – this is quite normal. Frequently a shade that might look correct can appear entirely different when it is actually applied to the skin. Involve them during the skin matching process: it may fascinate them that the product was either too yellow, pink or grey against their skin but, more importantly, involving them helps you to develop a rapport and it will empower them to make informed decisions for their preferred skin match colour and application technique.

Only a very small amount of camouflage crème or powder is needed to achieve a skin match.

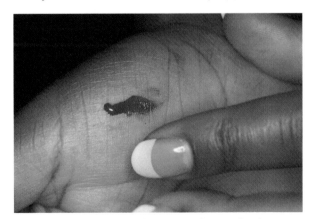

03 only an small amount is required

The most economical tool to remove the camouflage crème from its container is a cocktail stick. On no account should the cocktail stick ever be used as a spatula or directly on anyone or continued to be held by you – simply transfer the small amount off the stick onto your clean palm and discard the stick.

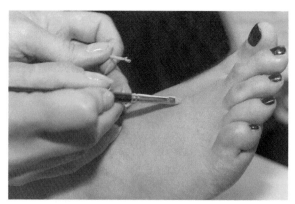

02 do not use the cocktail stick as a palette or hold it close to anyone (model kindly posed especially for this photograph)

Putting any form of palette against someone's skin is very impersonal, could cause injury or be perceived as a weapon. It also means that you will not see the product as clearly as you will when it is on your palm (palettes, spatulas and protective gloves could also distort the camouflage colour).

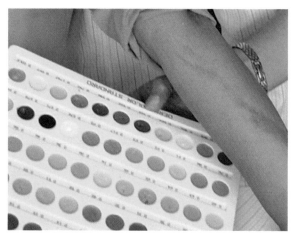

it is difficult to judge a skin match colour by holding a sample palette close to anyone (model kindly posed especially for this photograph)
© BASC Member 2160 (at Aniquem, Peru)

If the chosen camouflage product is powder format, then you will need to sprinkle (or spoon) a small amount from its container into your palm or onto a tissue. If you are using a stick camouflage or cosmetic concealer, then you will need to scrape off a small amount into your palm.

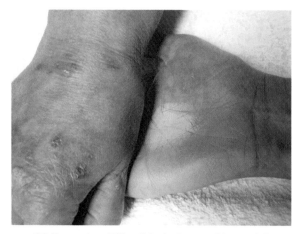

03 it can be difficult to judge a skin match by placing your palm close to anyone

Your palm is an ideal receptacle and the warmth of your skin makes camouflage crèmes easier to apply. If you need to judge the camouflage against the person's skin, using your open palm is not psychologically threatening; whereas there is a tendency to clench your fingers into a fist when using the back of your hand as palette and they will sense you pushing them away or a blow coming towards them!

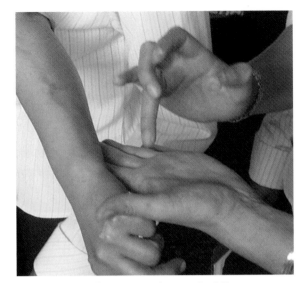

placing your palm against the person is non-threatening
© BASC Member 2160 (at Aniquem, Peru)

Choose a colour from the camouflage range that you think is similar or the same as the person's natural skin, remove a tiny amount and place it in your palm. Carefully spread the camouflage crème around with a clean finger.

During the skin matching process you will discover that it is easiest to use the pad of your finger. Your palm and finger can be kept clean by using wet-wipes and this will save your brushes and sponges being used during the skin match selection process.

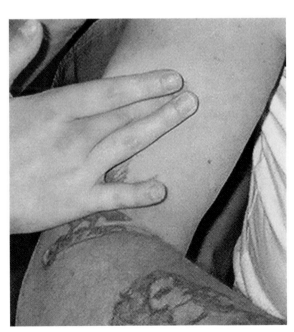

01 try to use the middle or ring ringer when applying camouflage

71

Avoid using the index finger as this unwittingly exerts pressure and can psychologically "point". Never press too hard as you can hurt people – even scars that are several years old can still be tender to the touch.

Using a finger, test by applying the product on the person's skin **beside** the scar or dermatosis to see if it is an acceptable skin match to them. Only apply to an area of skin no bigger than half the size of your little fingernail. If the area to be camouflaged is where embarrassment may be an issue, you can create the skin match colour on skin close by, and then guide them on how to apply the camouflage onto the required area when they return home. It is easier to apply camouflage to a knee or elbow which is flexed and to avoid any suggestion of a fist when working the back of a hand (and on knuckles) ask them to hold a wad of couch paper.

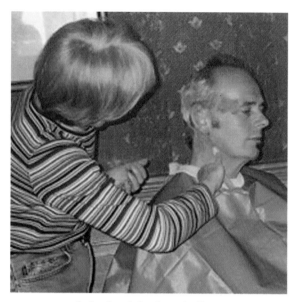

apply test patch close to the area
© BASC

If the initial or subsequent colour selection is not right, then you will have to remove the test patch and start again. Such trial and error can make the area requiring camouflage tender. If you believe the area is becoming sensitive, or erythema begins, then work elsewhere on the area requiring camouflage or on adjacent skin. This is vital for erythematic conditions (such as rosacea), otherwise the condition will become inflamed. Avoid applying the test patch over hyperkeratinised skin (such as psoriasis) because it will be difficult to totally remove any unacceptable colour from between the plaques.

Make a note of the unsuccessful colour, and move on to one that you consider a better match. Continue to make a note of all colours that you discount, otherwise you will end up going round in circles. A simple recording method is to return the cocktail stick to the colour just used – embed the clean, unused end in the camouflage crème – breaking the stick if the colour was unsuitable. Leave the stick unbroken if the colour was good but not fully acceptable. Using the cocktail stick as a record will also prevent any temptation to place the stick close to the person or retain it in your hand.

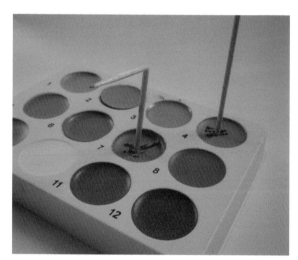

03 cocktail sticks in the palette
record tried colours

If you do have difficulty in achieving an acceptable skin match, and you sense that the person is weary of the procedure, arrange another consultation and say that it is **you** and **not** their skin that is at fault. Never, ever make any suggestion that it is impossible to create a skin match for them.

When you think that you have achieved a reasonable skin match, ask the person what they think. If there is any hesitation then try another skin tone close to the first and allow the person to decide which they believe is the better match.

If no single colour is a good match, then you will need to mix more than one colour together. Make a note of the ratio of the mix. Although this will not be a precise measurement, the person will need this information when ordering their products.

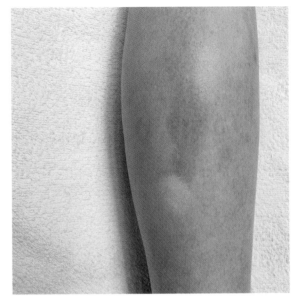

03 provide a selection of acceptable skin match for them to choose which one they prefer

It is **not** recommended that you mix more than two colours together otherwise the person will suppose their skin does not have a recognised colour matching crème or that the mixing process is too laborious. If you suggest a camouflage routine that will either take too long or require too much mixing of crèmes, then people may just give up and not do it.

Once you have agreed an acceptable skin colour match with them, you then need to demonstrate the preferred method of application.

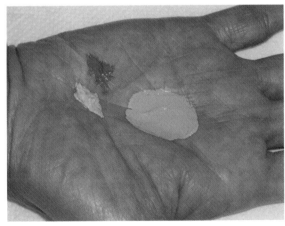

03 mixing two together to create acceptable match

application techniques

the appropriate application method will depend on the size and location of the area requiring camouflage. At the same time, you need to consider safe and comfortable working practices. It is important to remember that many dermatosis and scar tissue can be tender to the touch, (even painful) and some will be itchy. Whichever application method is chosen, you must apply sufficient pressure for the product to transfer to the person's skin but at the same time be gentle (so as not to hurt) while being careful not to tickle. There is a risk that the novice can lift the product back off the skin during the application, or apply too thin a layer; practice will eliminate either of those.

If your application technique appears to take too long, people will not attempt to use camouflage. You must advise them to use the method most comfortable for their needs and easiest to achieve, because your role also includes teaching them how to successfully apply their camouflage. Your application demonstration would be considered a failure if you use a method different to them.

Once these decisions have been made, camouflage one-third of the area. This will allow people to appraise 'before and after' application and observe the application technique.

Also, if you camouflaged the whole area straightaway, the person would have no opportunity to gauge how successful the camouflage is and have no area left to demonstrate their application technique. If seeing the camouflage free section is affecting the person's appraisal, the solution is to place a clean tissue over the non-camouflaged area.

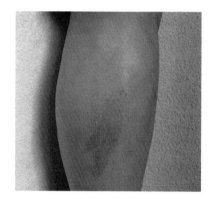

03 café a lait lesion with camouflage applied to top half only

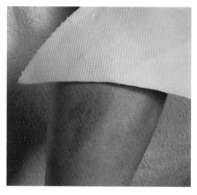

03 *upper half covered with tissue to show café au lait lesion*

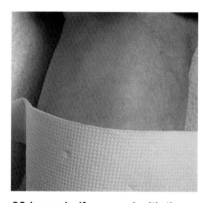

03 lower half covered with tissue to show camouflage area

Sometimes people can still 'see' their dermatosis, even when it has been successfully camouflaged. To illustrate this afterimage phenomenon, stare at figure 1 for 30 seconds and then immediately look at figure 2. Two things should happen - the colourless circle will now appear faintly coloured and the red image of figure 1 will surround figure 2.

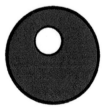

figure 1

figure 2

There is no instant formula that can be specified for any particular condition or brand of camouflage. Whatever method you choose, the camouflage must be applied sparingly and only to the skin requiring it. The reasons for this are,

- a more natural look can be achieved
- the outcome could be spoiled if the camouflage is extended too far over the surrounding skin

If you need to apply more than one layer of camouflage, then two (or even three) fine layers correctly set are more durable/stable on the skin than one thick application.

Camouflage is considered successful when there is minimal colour difference between the product and surrounding skin. If there is a margin it will be necessary for you to carefully blend the product away from the camouflaged area over the immediate surrounding skin.

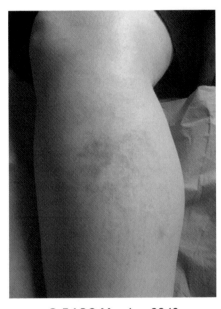

© BASC Member 2249
The British Association of Sclerotherapy

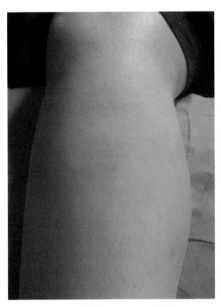

© BASC Member 2249
The British Association of Sclerotherapy

There are three effective methods for camouflage application. They are using,

- fingertips
- cosmetic brushes
- cosmetic sponges

Airbrushing might be an alternative method; this technique is discussed separately.

All application methods will give delicate to total coverage. Practise with each technique and assess the outcomes. You will discover that each method can affect the end result.

You will need to remove sufficient quantity from the chosen camouflage to achieve one-third coverage of the required area. Unless unavoidable, try not to include too much of the surrounding skin - keep the application to the area needing camouflage. Unless otherwise stated, the same process to transfer product from container to palm applies to all methods of application.

using fingertips
this can be done in several ways. With a clean finger, pick up the camouflage from your palm and,

press and roll
- best suited for small areas
- to blend camouflage margin into surrounding skin

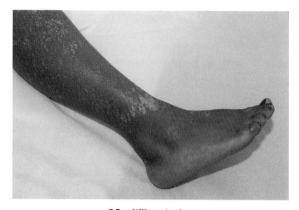

02 vitiligo to leg

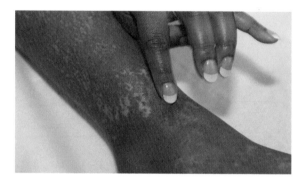

02 press and roll technique

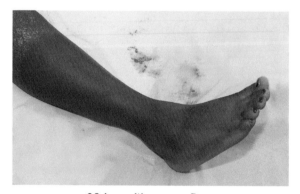

02 leg with camouflage

rub

- easiest for ears and joints
- over hyperkeratinised lesions
- over mesh grafts (when graft is over 1 year old)

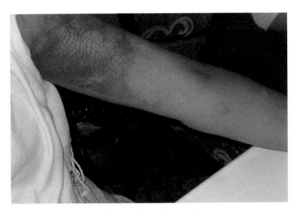

03 mesh skin graft

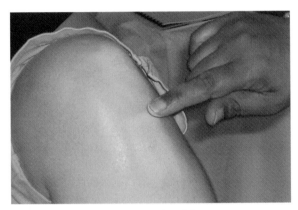

rubbing over bent knee
© BASC

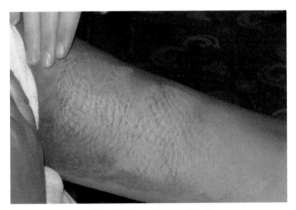

03 rubbing in method

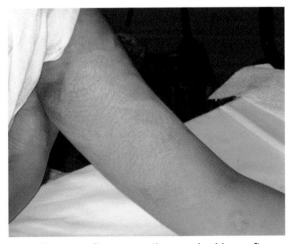

03 camouflage over the mesh skin graft

77

wiping using one or more fingertips

- the quickest method for larger areas
- more gentle over bruised-tender skin
- to blend camouflage margin into the surrounding skin

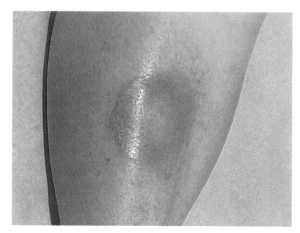

02 red lesion on leg

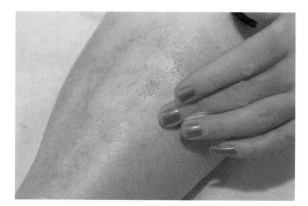

02 wiping technique

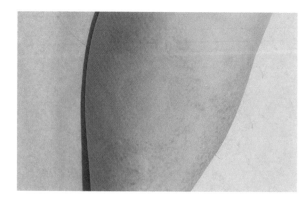

02 red lesion camouflaged

tap

- to blend margin into surrounding skin
- best suited when a second layer of camouflage is required

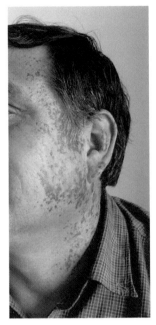

chloasma
© BASC Member 2160
(at Aniquem, Peru)

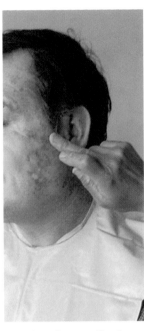

tapping method
© BASC Member 2160
(at Aniquem, Peru)

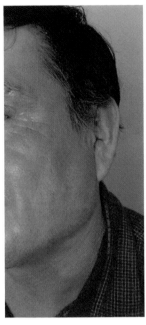

camouflage over the chloasma
© BASC Member 2160
(at Aniquem, Peru)

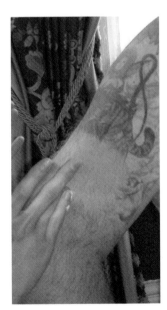

*carefully tapping on the skin
match does not dislodge the
complementary layer*

Experience shows that people will generally choose to use their fingers to apply their camouflage. Using fingertips reduces cost implications (for both you and them) and eliminates the hygiene requirement of cleaning brushes and sponges after each use; also it is a simple routine for the person to wash their hands before applying their camouflage.

using a brush

the brush must be clean and dry and a suitable width so it does not go onto the surrounding skin. Brushes are best used for small patches requiring camouflage and, irrespective of the size of the brush, are too laborious to use over larger areas. Always use a brush for,

- narrow scars
- creating lip shape
- creating eyebrow hairs
- when working close to eyelash area

Brushes are also useful for dotting concealer (or camouflage) along dark lines around the eye before carefully blending with sponge, brush or fingertip.

Pick up the camouflage from your palm and gently stroke the brush over the area. You may find that on narrow scars it is better to work in an 'S' or 'Z' pattern along the scar, rather than using a continual line. Following application with a brush, you may need to use one of the fingertip methods to blur any hard edges and to blend the camouflage into the surrounding skin.

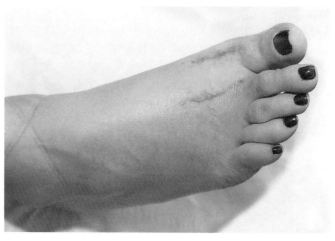

02 narrow scar on foot

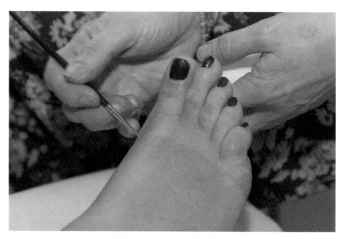

02 brush application

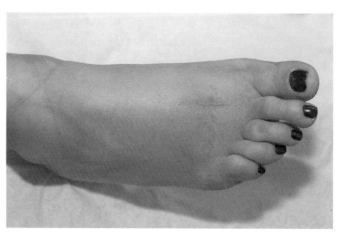

02 scar with camouflage

using a sponge

is best over very delicate skin. Using a clean wedge (or sponge), pick up the camouflage from your palm and wipe (or use a press and roll motion) over the required area.

The side of a wedge is ideal for feathering camouflage onto the surrounding skin – blur any hard edges with a fingertip.

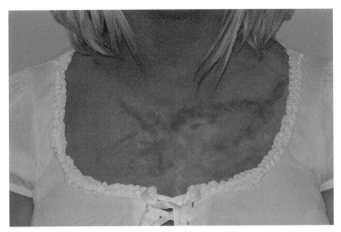

01 scald injury (sustained as a child) – following medical procedures, the scarring is flat to surrounding skin

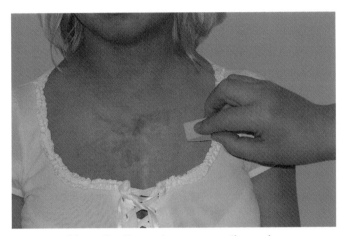

01 application using a cosmetic wedge

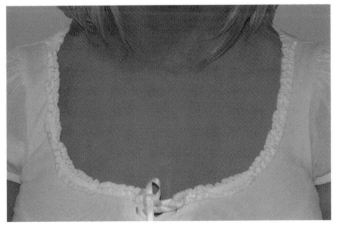

01 with camouflage applied

setting the camouflage

after applying the camouflage crème by the selected method, and blending into the immediate surrounding skin, it needs to be set with loose powder. There is no need to set powder camouflage, airbrush inks and some liquid camouflage products with loose powder.

If you use more than one layer of crème then you must set the layer before applying the second or subsequent layers, otherwise you will end up with one thick layer, which will not be stable on the skin and will look contrived. You must set a complementary layer before applying the skin match to prevent the colours intermixing on the skin.

The secret to successful setting is to apply powder over the camouflage crème. This can be achieved by loading your powder puff and rolling it over the crème. Alternatively, you can sprinkle directly from 'salt cellar' or 'pepper pot' style containers and press the powder into the crème with the puff. Take care, especially when working on the face, not to create 'clouds' of powder that could irritate eyes and lungs. The best method to prevent this is to load the puff with powder and then fold it on itself and carefully rub the powder into the fibre. While it may appear that the powder has now been absorbed by the puff, when you apply the puff onto the skin the powder will transfer.

Press into the crème, wait a minute or two to allow the crème to absorb the powder, then with a clean powder brush (or the reverse or side of the puff) flick off any powder that has not been absorbed. If you have applied too much powder it will eventually cake as the skin warms up.

Briskly brushing to and fro over naturally hirsute areas will remove any camouflage that has attached to vellus hair.

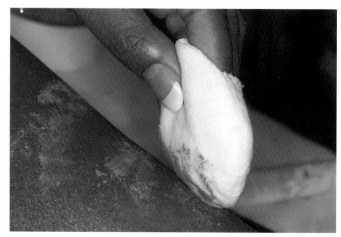

02 setting the camouflage crème with loose powder

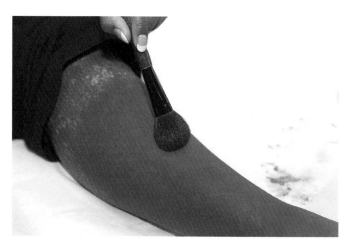

02 brush off excess

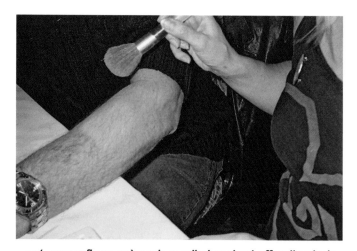

set camouflage crème is easily brushed off vellus hair

fixing spray will increase stability/durability of all camouflage products (especially sealing a complementary colour or a first layer of camouflage) and gives the area a natural radiance. It is better to apply a very fine layer of fixing spray at first then build it up to match the sheen of the surrounding skin. If you overdo it, you will have to take the camouflage off and start again!

If your decision includes using a fixing spray, then follow the manufacturer's guidelines on facial and body application. It is not recommended that you, or anyone, sprays fixing products onto the face, head or cape area. For those areas, you need to spray a small amount of fixing into your clean palm, pick up the product with a dry wedge and pat it over the camouflage. The fixing will take a few seconds to dry. If required, apply a second or third layer – build up the product carefully to the desired result.

You can spray fixing onto limbs and trunk, holding the container at the manufacturer's recommended distance (and angle) from the skin. Should the fixing give sheen when a matt look is preferred, then simply apply a fine layer of loose powder over the fixing.

blotting with a damp sponge cloth
this may not be an essential part of people's routine, but when required you will need a clean cloth for each person. Dampen the cloth with clean, warm water and carefully place it over the powdered crème camouflage. Press gently, otherwise you may move the camouflage, and carefully lift the cloth away from the skin.

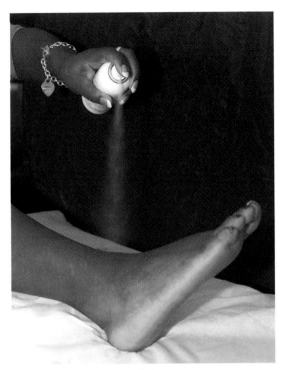

02 using fixing spray

stippling and faking faults

creating an acceptable skin camouflage will make the underlying problem less visible, but having a "perfect patch of skin" may still draw attention to the area. The solution is to "fake faults" by recreating natural discolouration. The addition of freckles, appropriate veins, broken capillaries, beard shadow and the occasional mole will make the solid skin match merge into the surrounding skin and be totally camouflaged. However, faking faults is not automatically required and must be considered as an option only to be used when needed, such as for symmetry or breaking up a large area of camouflage.

All your artistic skills come into action here – you will need to reproduce exactly what you can see in the surrounding skin (or mirror what presents the opposite side of the face, trunk or limb); but do remember, less is always best! involve them, especially when deciding if faked faults are required.

A better result is achieved when you apply faked faults onto the camouflage crème <u>before</u> it has been powdered. Once the fault has been applied, tap very lightly over it with the ball of your finger to sink it into the skin match. This will make it appear as natural as those present in the uncamouflaged skin. Then set with powder and complete the consultation.

application techniques
the method required will depend on the fault you need to recreate. Pick up the selected colour and place it in the palm of your hand, just as you would with skin coloured camouflage

using a stipple sponge
pick up colour on the sponge and test for depth of colour on your palm or sheet of couch paper. This will ensure no error is made when the stipple is used on the person. If you stipple directly onto them, and it proves to be an incorrect colour or too much product (because the sponge is overloaded), then you will need to remove all of the underlying camouflage and begin again.

In a single movement lightly roll the stipple across the area while trying not to smudge the underlying camouflage. Care must be taken not to create a 'rubber stamp' effect. Start with sparse stippling where it is needed, building up the faked fault until it matches the surrounding skin.

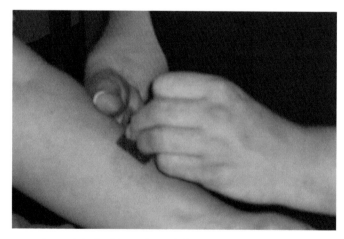

try not to "rubber stamp" the sponge on the skin
© BASC

to create beard shadow

you may need to add a tiny amount of blue to create very dark blue-black shadows (use your palm as the mixing palette)

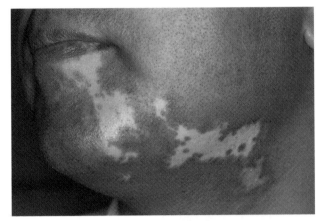

02 leucoderma to beard shadow area

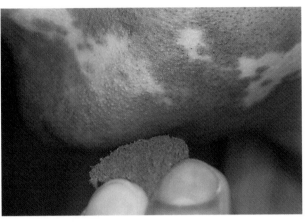

02 stippling beard shadow

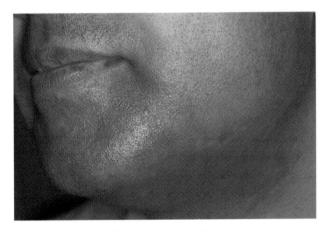

02 shadow applied

to create abundant freckles

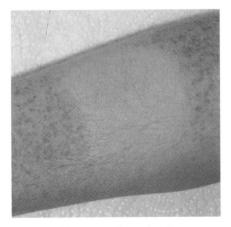

03 camouflaged skin

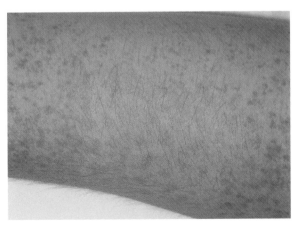

03 multiple freckles applied

to create thread veins and broken capillaries

in this example the camouflage was created by stippling erythema – no skin match camouflage was applied beneath.

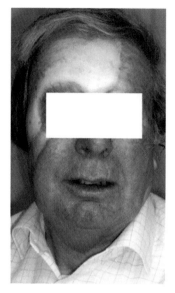

skin graft
© BASC Member 1022

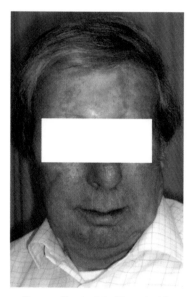

camouflage stippled (without skin match foundation) to mimic florid complexion
© BASC Member 1022

using a stipple sponge to create a delicate skin match

in this example the person preferred to apply the skin match stippled to the area

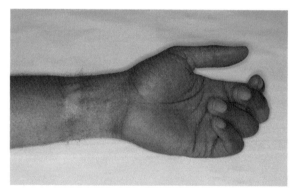

02 hypopigmentation to wrist

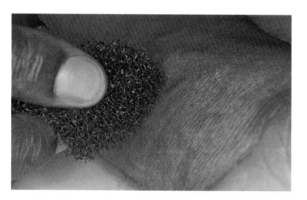

02 skin match applied using the stipple sponge

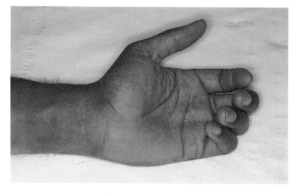

02 finished result

using a brush or cotton bud

you can create sporadic moles, occasional freckles and even age-spots! You will achieve a better result if you vary the size and shape. Always mimic the surrounding skin, some may require more than others,

to create moles

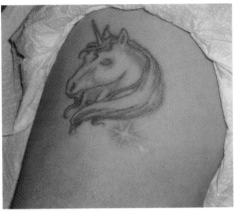

03 tattoo

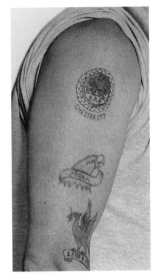

01 tattoo

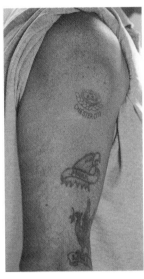

01 half of tattoo with camouflage and several moles applied

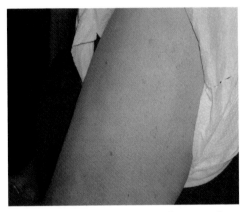

03 skin matched camouflage and occasional moles applied

to create veins

try not to create long straight lines: a broken line and feint impression of a vein will be more convincing,

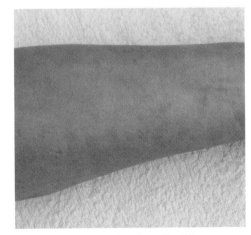

03 fake vein running length of inner arm

There will be occasions when you need to recreate a facial feature (partially or full shape), such as lips and eyebrows.

shaping and defining lips

first agree with the person the lip colour and shape, and their preferred product (camouflage crème or lip staining pen). It might help to outline the shape (using a decorative cosmetic lip liner or contrasting colour crème camouflage) just outside the intended margin of the lips – then simply infil with the chosen product. This is especially important when working with lip stains. Once the camouflage or stain is set, the outline can be removed using a cotton bud dipped in cleansing lotion. If you use the lip staining products to draw the lip shape, then a specialist pen remover (or alcohol wipe) will dislodge any errors. Lips created with camouflage crème will need powdering – which might make the lips appear unnaturally matt. The application of a lipstick sealer (available from chemists and beauty counters) will prolong the stability of the camouflage, and some will create a semi-matt finish. For those without lips, the long-term solution may be medical tattooing.

Some people may prefer to use their fingertip when applying their lips, but for hygienic reasons you should always use a brush on people's lips. When applying any product onto someone else's lips it is best to work quickly, efficiently and without tickling. Feathering with the brush will tickle the lips: the moment you remove the brush the person will invariably scratch their lips (usually with their teeth) – removing most of what you have applied! People's lips need to be closed and not pulled into an 'apple' or 'letterbox' shape.

Place the crème camouflage in the palm of your hand and using a brush suitable to the mouth size, pick up sufficient product to complete the application. Never return the brush to the product in its container once contact has been made with the lips. You will need to replace the felt tip of pen format lip stains between use.

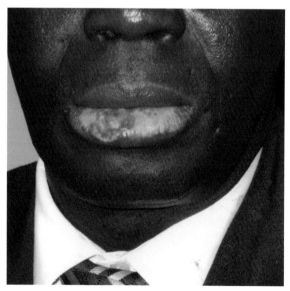

hypopigmentation to lower lip
© BASC Member 1022

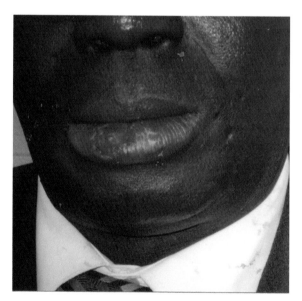

lip stain outcome
© BASC Member 1022

application technique in eight continuous strokes!

it does not matter whether you start with the top or the bottom lip, but you will find it easier working from the corner of the mouth and stop at the middle of the lip; you should never apply in one continuous movement across the whole length of the lip because you will distort the mouth shape as you go along. It may help if you keep your little finger firmly in the centre of the chin to allow you to work swiftly without moving your hand away from the face.

It is easier if you create the outline first, which is achieved by holding the fine edge of the brush on the lip. Remember not to feather – use bold continuous sweeps with the brush.

outline in four brush strokes

upper lip - working from one corner to the centre then opposite corner to centre – repeat same movement for lower lip

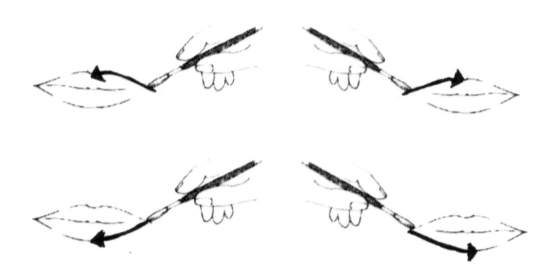

arrows indicate the brush or lip stain direction

infil in four brush strokes

now twist the brush in your fingers to work flat side on and repeat the same four movements to infil the lip.

problem solving

- if there is a drooped outline to the mouth, apply a little skin match camouflage over the drooping area, then redraw the contour line to match the unaffected side
- if the person wants to wear lipstick, it is better to use either lip stains instead of camouflage or long-lasting lipstick over the sealed camouflage. Most cosmetic houses have a range of lipsticks that are designed to be longer lasting than normal lipsticks
- lip stains may be a better option for anyone having maxillofacial or reconstructive surgery to their lip area, or for those who have excessive saliva
- if there is no prospect of reconstructive surgery, the long-term solution may be to have the lips recreated by medical tattoo

shaping and defining eyebrows

whether it is angled, sloping, curved or straight in shape depends on the existing shape of the brow and people's preference. However, if the brow hairs have been over-tweezed or no longer grow due to a medical condition or procedure, you can help the person devise a suitable eyebrow shape that is appropriate to the contour of their eye.

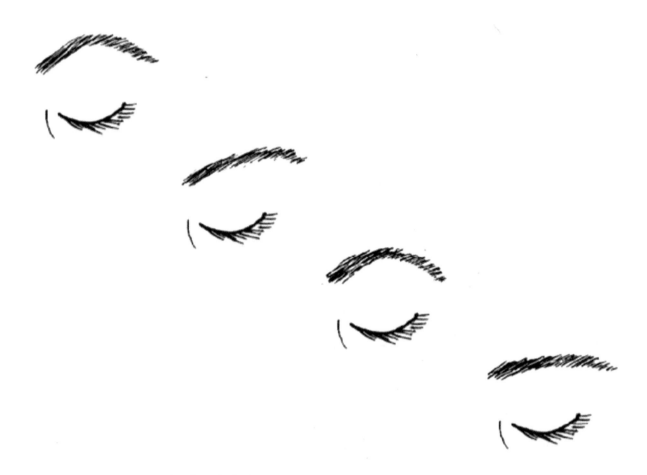

example of angled, sloping, curved and straight brow shapes

As a general rule, a very round prominent eye will benefit from an angled or straight brow, rather than a curved brow, which would emphasise the eye shape. A gentle curved eyebrow will enhance almond shaped eyes, whereas the angled or straight brow creates a hard look to that shaped eye. Some, especially males, will prefer a straight or slightly sloping brow shape.

Always confirm the eyebrow shape, colour and density with the person, especially when the chosen product is a staining pen.

eyebrow position

the eyebrow should extend between (a) and (b), the apex should be just past the iris (c).

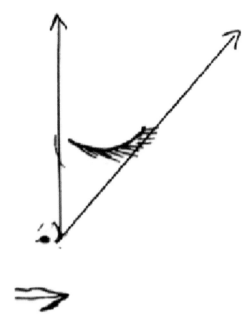

extend between (a) and (b)

Explain to the person how you will be using the eyebrow brush (or similar straight applicator) to confirm the brow position and apex. It may help to carefully mark the start, apex and finishing points (using the same colour agreed for the brow hairs).

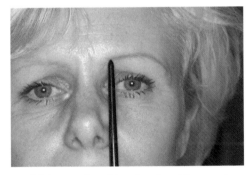

02 brow should not extend beyond point horizontal to nostril (a)

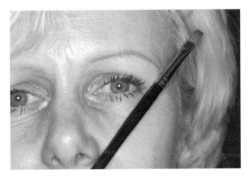

02 brow should not extend beyond point oblique to nostril (b)

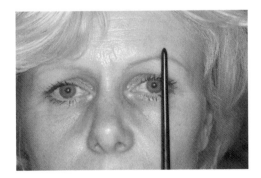

02 apex just past the iris (c)

product choice

skin stains and waterproof products should be taken into consideration for people whose medical condition or lifestyle might make the eyebrow streak or run, and may prove to be the better choice for children and males. Decorative cosmetic eyebrow products are sold in pencil and liquid format; you can also achieve a natural looking result if you use eye shadow. For those who have no eyebrow hair, the long-term solution may be medical tattooing.

A taupe colour works best for fair, auburn and grey haired people; mid to dark brown will give natural colouring to brunettes. Black can be too harsh and ageing unless, of course, that is the natural hair and brow colour.

application technique

advise the person to keep their forehead expressionless, and not distort the skin when applying the product. Pressing too firmly, or using a harsh product could disturb any camouflage application. Build up the depth and length of the brow carefully.

To achieve realistic brows, use short strokes that mimic natural hair growth, rather than a continual line and then carefully blend it in to achieve a soft and very natural eyebrow. If too much is applied, the excess can be removed with a cotton-bud.

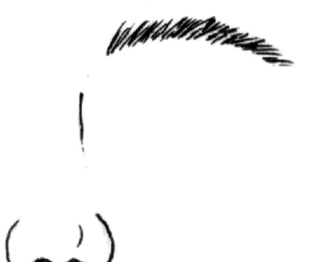

reaffirming the skin camouflage application sequence

problem solving is included at the end of this chapter, however, most difficulties occur when the novice practitioner forgets the sequence of application which is,

confirm your understanding

first of all, always try the agreed skin colour match to see if that will give sufficient cover. If it does, proceed accordingly and complete the consultation

if it is not sufficient to cover, but is beginning to camouflage

then apply powder and press it into the crème. Wait for the powder to be absorbed and then remove excess with a brush (or blot with a damp sponge), then try a second layer of the skin tone colour match. If that then gives sufficient cover, apply powder and complete the consultation

if a dark shadow is still visible

then you will need to use the complementary colour theory,

- wipe off the skin colour match and apply the complementary colour and powder. Wait for the powder to be absorbed and then remove excess
- if the complementary colour blocks out the hyperpigmentation with no shadow showing through, then apply the skin match and powder and complete the consultation
- if the complementary is showing through the skin match, then it will be necessary to apply a second layer of skin match. If that then gives sufficient cover, apply powder and complete the consultation

When the camouflaged area needs natural imperfections (faking faults) added, then apply these over the skin match, set the camouflage and complete the consultation.

above all, remember to keep it simple – do not over-complicate the process!

confirm people's understanding

the final phase is to gauge whether people understand the application process by asking them to cover the remaining area that needs camouflage. This will give you the chance to confirm and affirm the application process and make any suggestions to ensure that the camouflage is applied correctly.

Show people how to use their palm as a palette, for the reasons mentioned earlier, and always let them use their preferred method when they demonstrate the application technique back to you. Don't forget to offer them a wet-wipe to clean the palm of their hand and fingers before applying the product.

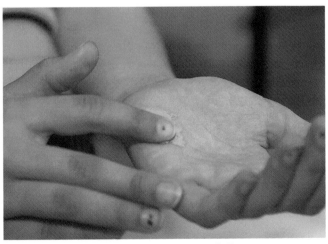

02 using palm as a palette

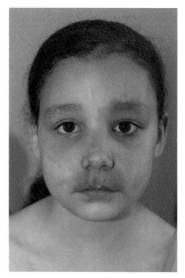
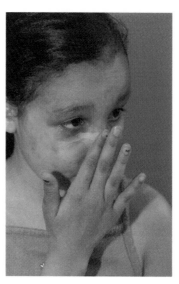
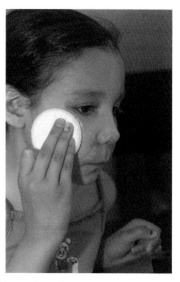

02 before camouflage application

02 demonstrating their preferred method of application

02 setting the crème with powder

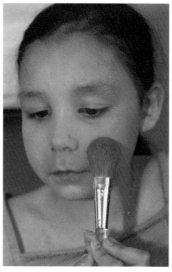
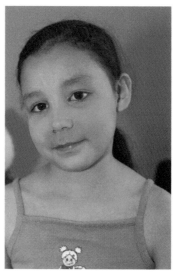

02 brushing off excess powder

02 camouflage application complete

Before finalising the consultation you need to make certain that the person,

- is happy with the camouflage products used
- has agreed the camouflage colour is an acceptable match
- knows how to apply the camouflage
- if required, knows how to apply any faked faults
- is aware of products and actions which may accidentally dislodge or remove the camouflage
- knows how to remove the camouflage
- is aware that their doctor should be advised that camouflage products are being applied so their medical notes can be updated
- knows where to obtain the products

People will be reassured to know that they can return to you for another consultation should their skin change colour or because they wish to consider alternative colours or formulations.

camouflage application to post mortem skin

this specialist section is aimed at mortuary technicians, embalmers and those who prepare the deceased for viewing within funeral directors' premises to use when camouflage becomes a compassionate act to alleviate distress.

There are two circumstances when there may be a need to apply products to post mortem skin:
-   within a mortuary, for identification purposes
-   within funeral directors, for final viewing

The process of bereavement and saying goodbye is emotional and traumatic. This is especially so when the death is unexpected, such as a road traffic accident or violence. Identification is required for Coroner or forensic/police needs. It is distressing for the bereaved to be made aware of the cause of death and it is insensitive for that to remain evident. Camouflage application usually involves only the face, neck and hands; it is not necessary to apply to skin hidden by clothing or shroud. Although it would be inappropriate to apply camouflage to putrefied skin, the skin will be in the initial stages of autolysis (cell-tissue decomposition) and rigor mortis (which starts about three hours after death and lasts approximately thirty-six) evidence of which may be present. The skin will feel cold and clammy; post embalming the skin will be drier. The skin will be malleable pre and post rigor mortis, but immobile following the embalming process.

All camouflage applied must withstand the natural changes in body temperature as well as ambient fluctuations between refrigeration, viewing room and open casket environments. Camouflage should resemble the natural skin colour and mimic how the deceased preferred their image to be. This may require you to recreate their dermatosis, such as a port wine stain or vitiligo, or to apply decorative cosmetics. All applications must be minimal, giving a delicate hint of the desired image. The bereaved will understand that the person's skin has less colour and appreciate a suggestion rather than vivid healthy cosmetic skin colours. Blusher is not required! Always request a photograph that will give a good indication of hairstyle and any make-up worn.

identification of skin colour

the variations within each skin classification group become less obvious, which simplifies skin colour matching. The absence of vascular circulation will present a pallid and ashen pallor to the upper part of the body and lividity (liver mortis) as dark discolouration where the blood supply has settled. Lividity can also suggest bruising, which will be psychologically disturbing to the bereaved. The embalming process can eliminate liver mortis.

Additional discolouration may be due to the circumstances causing death, such as heavily jaundiced skin from drugs and chemotherapy, gravel from road traffic accident, carbon from an explosion, greenish skin stains (due to drowning), acid burns from vomit, as well as the physical effects of violence. However discoloured, a complementary colour is rarely required under the skin match.

product choice

a water-in-oil (crème) product will survive better than other forms of skin camouflage. It may be necessary to dilute and further soften the crème camouflage with specialist products to prevent any drag over the skin, especially when "skin-slip" is present or the skin is exceptionally fragile. In such instances it will also be necessary to use the fixing spray as a skin primer. Loose powder will be needed to set the camouflage, but be careful not to over apply as it could cake or turn the crème into a paste. Fixing spray to give semi or full sheen to the skin can be applied over the set camouflage.

application technique

test the suggested skin match on an area of skin that will not be visible. The testing sequence is identical to that previously mentioned. Using a cotton bud instead of the pad of your finger to apply the test patch will minimalise wasting protective gloves.

Whether you then apply your selected skin match by brush, cosmetic sponge or with (gloved) fingers will depend on the stability and condition of the skin. Apply powder in the same method as for living skin.

Air brushing is not a recommended method because the product choice is less compatible with post mortem skin.

Application of "faked faults" (including beard shadow) follows that already mentioned. You can use skin stains or camouflage crème to recreate lips and seal the product with fixing spray.

It may be that a relative or member of the community will request to apply any cosmetics over the camouflage, or prefer to assist with the laying-out process. You will need to discuss with them whether skin camouflage should be applied prior to their involvement.

other considerations

before you begin, you will also need to gain permission from the Pathologist (Coroner or Police) that your actions will not interfere with legal proceedings.

There may be occasions when you need to conceal trauma (and visible sutures) to the skin to give it an undamaged texture. Skin plastic and specialist silicone can be used to good effect here. You will need to seal the plug with a layer of super-glue to both keep the plug in position and create a skin primer to accept the crème camouflage.

Super-glue is the preferred choice when applying eyelashes – other glues will just not adhere to the skin. Measure the lash strip and cut to size; confirm if you need to distress the lashes to match natural growth. Apply a fine line of glue to the required area and using tweezers hold the lash strip in place until the glue cures. Skin staining pens can be used to recreate missing eyebrow hairs.

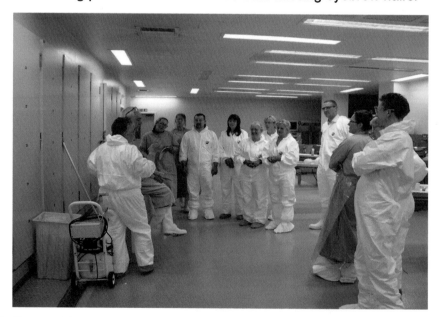

due to the sensitive nature, BASC felt it prudent not to include before/after photographs of camouflage application to post mortem skin.
this photograph was taken during the Specialist Training event 2009 at the Mortuary, RLUH
© BASC Member 2319, Mortuary, RLUH

using an airbrush

when using airbrush equipment, it is vital that you comply with the manufacturer's application and safety instructions – especially the air volume (CFM) and air pressure (PSI). Additional safety precautions you and people need to be aware of are to,

- protect clothing and surrounding surfaces – which may include the chair, table, carpet and even wall – as the airbrushing system creates a fine mist of colour!
- work in a ventilated room and do not inhale the mist (wear a nose-mouth mask if your environment contravenes these safety precautions)

airbrush inks

as with all camouflage products, a little airbrush ink goes a long way. Some inks dry almost immediately on application; those containing silicone take slightly longer to dry.

It would be too time-consuming and wasteful to load the airgun container with ink until you have created an acceptable skin match. The easiest method is to proceed in the same way as you would with traditional camouflage. Put a small dot of the colour from the bottle into the clean palm of your hand, pick it up with your fingertip and apply it over a small area of skin requiring the camouflage. If there is no acceptable skin match within the colours, then the inks can be mixed in the palm of your hand. Once the skin match is achieved and agreed with them you can then mix the inks in a spare container and load the airgun. Density can be built up by applying subsequent layers.

It is not recommended, for hygienic reasons, to return any unused ink to its original container. The airbrush will need to be cleaned thoroughly before working with either another colour or on another.

When working on a person's face and neck, you must advise them to close their eyes and hold their breath. This will, of course, make self-application an almost impossible task for them! Your role is to achieve an application that is appropriate for the person to manage - which makes using airbrushing equipment not a practicable choice. The simple solution is for people to use the ink in the same way as normal camouflage and ignore the airbrush equipment altogether!

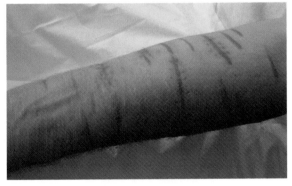

self harm scarring
© BASC Member 2303

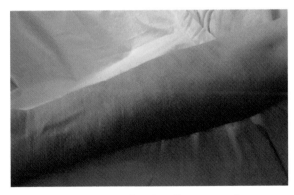

*application result using the camouflage
without the airbrush equipment*
© BASC Member 2303

Some people find the colours premixed in aerosols to be a quick and efficient way to cover hypopigmentation and hyper-pigmentation and scarring to body and limbs. Although the colour range will be limited, this format has proved successful when initially introducing camouflage to people who self harm.

Attending a salon for airbrushing, or using an aerosol to self apply faux tanning products may also be an option for people to consider.

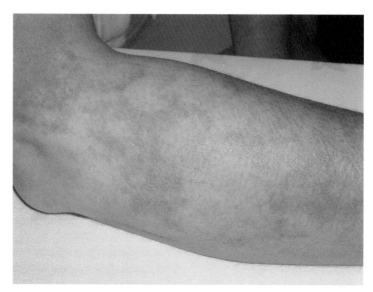

03 vitiligo

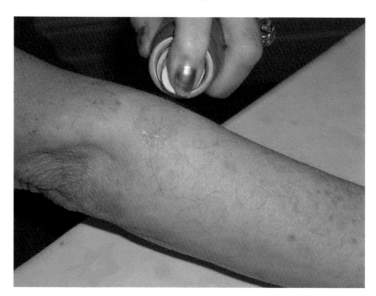

03 application using an aerosol camouflage

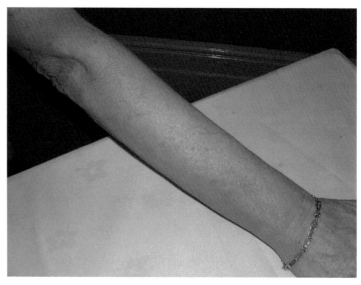

03 camouflage result

faux tan products

the following general principles apply to crème, mousse, and liquid faux tan products, for both your information and to advise people who may later use this method themselves. People may prefer to self-apply or attend their beauty/spa salon for applications.

A patch test must be carried out 24 hours before full application to confirm there is no allergic reaction. The test patch also allows the person to judge the depth of colour achieved by one application.

Most brands require you to exfoliate the skin before applying the product (usually this is included with their kit). Any hair removal (depilation and epilation) must be done at least 24 hours before the patch test. Contraindications are identical to those for camouflage applications, plus the cessation of any IPL or LASER treatment.

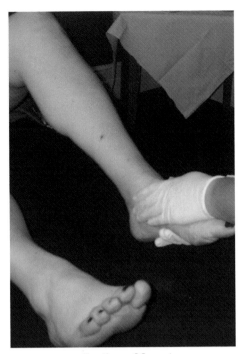

application of faux tan
© BASC

application technique

apply a barrier cream, such as petroleum jelly (or the emollient supplied with the kit) to the naturally pigmented margin of skin where it meets the hypopigmented. This will prevent the product from accidentally staining non-leucoderma (and vitiligo) areas and prevent any dark halo where the two areas of skin meet. Unfortunately there is a risk that any natural hyperpigmented lesions, such as solar lentigo, will darken in colour.

Using the product at its full strength, apply the faux tan with a brush (or by your fingertips protected by gloves) only to the depigmented skin. If using an airbrush to apply the faux tan, then it may prove difficult not to cover larger areas of skin. Some brands then require you to gently massage the product on the skin, stopping when the product turns a different texture or colour. Explain that the colour now seen is not the finished tan, and that any streakiness should not affect the end result.

Allow the product to dry – this can take five to ten minutes depending on brand used. Once the area has dried, buff the product off with a soft mitt or flannel.

Some brands suggest washing off any excess product immediately after this stage, others recommend that the tan is left to develop for several hours or overnight before washing. People might require subsequent applications to build up the colour to an acceptable match.

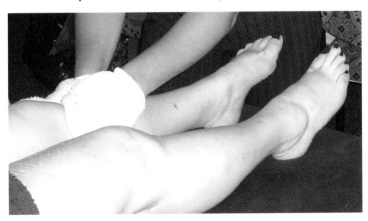

buffing the faux tan with flannel mitts
© BASC

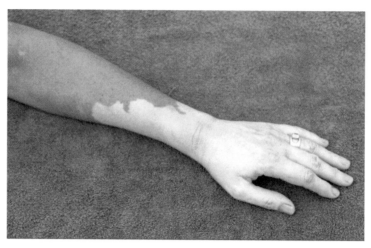

vitiligo
© Alida DePase BASC Member 2158

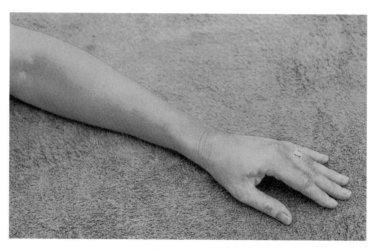

camouflage using faux tan
© Alida DePase BASC Member 2158

If required, people can also apply half strength faux tan to the whole area, such as their arms, or to their whole body and face to give an even "tan" effect.

People will need to top up their faux tan every week (consult manufacturer's guidelines for frequency). Some people find that after 4 to 5 weeks they need to stop their application and resume after a 2 to 3 week break to prevent any excessive or unnatural build-up of colour.

For reasons previously outlined, airbrushing is not a recommended self-application method, especially for faux tan to the face and neck. However, airbrushing faux tan is a very successful treatment provided by beauty therapists. A patch test applies.

Skin camouflage can be applied to faux tanned skin once the colour has fully developed and the skin has been cleansed of residue product.

a simple solution often solves a problem

camouflaged skin appears blanched on a photograph
camouflage crèmes, powders and setting powders containing reflective and whitening minerals (such as titanium dioxide) can "flash back white" on a photographic image.

- this is less likely to happen with photographs taken in daylight, or without the flash activated
- check the ingredients list and use alternative brands that do not contain the minerals
- you can minimalise the effect by applying a fine layer of decorative foundation (that also does not contain the minerals) over the camouflage crème

camouflaged skin sometimes has a grey-blue shadow
this may occur to erythematous lesions (such as rosacea, port wine stains, psoriasis) and scars when a person moves from a warm to a cold environment. This might cause a dilemma and people may need to consider which would be the most appropriate camouflage to use under these circumstances.

- apply a yellow/orange complementary (depending on skin group) under the skin matching camouflage
- apply a yellow/orange tinted powder (depending on skin group) to set the skin match

camouflage is difficult to spread
- some brands suggest priming the area with a fine application of moisturiser or sunblock – this gives some 'slip' when spreading the camouflage
- check that the product is not out of date and has dried out – throw away such products and buy a replacement
- ensure the skin is comfortably warm, which will make application easier
- if using a spatula, convert to using the palm method to hold the product as the palm will gently warm the crème
- reappraise the brand of camouflage being used and method of application – perhaps they are not suitable
- check that you are not applying the product too thickly

camouflage spreads too thinly
- remove excess oil (caused either by skin condition, residue from cleanser, camouflage crème, moisturiser) from the skin with a a gentle skin toner
- ensure application equipment is dry and, if using a damp sponge, that it is not too wet
- reappraise the brand of camouflage being used and the method of application – perhaps they are not suitable
- check that you are applying sufficient product to the area

camouflage spreads too thickly
- reappraise application method and brand being used
- dilute the camouflage crème with a product specially designed to do this

camouflage slides off the area
- this can happen over stretched or swollen skin and especially so over skin grafts. There are special priming products available that help to keep the camouflage adhered to the specified area. Apply a fine layer of primer, then continue with the camouflage application as usual. To some degree, moisturisers and sunscreen products will act as a primer as will a fine application of fixing spray before and under the camouflage
- the person's skin has excessive sebum or there is a residue of oil from the cleansing product. In either case, wipe over the area with a gentle toner and then apply the camouflage

camouflage now covers a larger area than needed or looks contrived
- always keep the camouflage application to the immediate area and carefully blend the margin between natural coloured skin

- remove excess camouflage with cleanser
- the addition of faked faults may solve the problem

skin match was good until it was powdered
- sometimes, especially for those with a suntan and skin groups 4 to 6, application of a brown-toned or bronzing powder will solve any problems where the skin match is good but is lacking a natural sheen
- if the camouflaged area appears chalky, then applying another brand of powder should solve the problem as it could be that the original product contains too much French chalk, talc, iron oxide or titanium dioxide
- powders that have a rice base are good at keeping the camouflage matt without any chalky or greying effects
- a coloured powder will change the skin match colour

camouflage appears too matt
if the camouflaged area needs to look semi-matt or have a full sheen then

- apply fixing spray
- try a fine application of bronzing powder over the set camouflage

camouflage appears too grey on the skin
if the camouflage appears too grey on the skin, then you may have chosen the incorrect base colour in the product to suit the base tone in their skin.

- in the case of sun-tanned and skin groups 4 to 6, make sure a mineral such as titanium dioxide is not the product's major ingredient

camouflage appears to go orange on the skin
if the camouflage appears to go orange on the skin, then you have chosen the incorrect base colour in the product to suite the base tone in their skin.

BASC is unaware of any medical or scientific evidence to support the hypothesis that "cosmetics can change colour due to the skin's acidity". Although skin with more pigment tends to be slightly more acidic, this would be insufficient to make any colour change.

camouflage appears "caked"
if you have applied too much powder it will eventually cake as the skin warms up, and applying too much around the eye area will emphasise any uneven texture to the skin.

Usually this is because the area has been over-worked or too much product has been applied. Remedy by removing and applying the product correctly, such as

- a fine (not thick) layer of camouflage crème is applied
- powder is patted over the area
- press the powder into the camouflage crème
- wait a minute or two
- brush off excess
- blot with damp sponge flannel

camouflage rubs off quickly or requires extra protection because of its location
- set with powder and then apply fixing spray
- use faux tan under the camouflage
- suggest that they do not scratch or rub the camouflaged skin (some people do this without realising they have a habit)
- if camouflage is to back of hands or fingers, then suggest that they take extra care when washing and drying their hands

dark circles around the eyes

people will find exactly where the camouflage (or concealer) needs to be placed if they point their chin towards their chest with their eyes looking into a mirror at eye level. You will also be able to place camouflage accurately when the person has their chin downward and you stand

-   you may find dark circles are difficult to block out unless a complementary colour is applied before the skin match. Dark circles around the eyes usually have blue-green undertones – you may find that a pale cream colour on skin groups 1 to 3, a peach colour for groups 4 to 5, and a terracotta colour for group 6, are useful complementary colours to try

halos and shadows to scars

make-up artists follow the rule that "light brings forward and dark takes back" when applying cosmetics to give extra contour to a face and glamorise facial features. However, medical graphic artists can use tattoo inks to create a nipple using trompe l'oeil. The idea of blending a slightly darker shade of camouflage to the highest part of keloid and hypertrophic scars, and applying a slightly lighter colour to the deepest part of atrophic scars, may make the scar seem slightly flatter when viewed from the front. However, the scar will not have that illusion when viewed at any other angle and if the blending is not 100% accurate the scar could appear bigger, higher or deeper

halos and shadows to dermatoses

although you have created an acceptable skin match, the skin surrounding the camouflaged area now appears lighter or darker, giving the camouflaged area a halo or shadow. To minimalise these effects stipple or blend the skin match carefully over the halo

If a dark halo remains visible, which can be the case with vitiligo and raised dermatoses, then you may need to apply a cream coloured camouflage first to the rim of the natural pigmented area, then the skin match over the whole. This will soften the difference between the camouflage, halo and the surrounding skin

The same principle applies to pale coloured halos – apply a darker coloured product under the skin match

If the halo or shadow remains visible, you will need to consider applying a complementary colour under the skin match

legs
-   if the camouflage looks contrived, you can add a very thin coat of the skin match over the whole leg, which will help blend back the camouflage
-   for larger areas requiring camouflage, you will have to treat the other leg in the same way to give both legs the same appearance
-   using a fixing spray over the set camouflage will give a natural sheen and make the camouflage more durable

An alternative to consider is using a faux tan, which may give a better and more lasting result

tattoos

if the tattoo remains visible, and the complementary and skin colours are correct, try sealing each layer with fixing spray

If the tattoo remains visible, your complementary colour has been incorrect

If the tattoo remains visible, and the complementary colour is correct, apply a second layer of complementary and/or two layers of skin match

*a quick tour of skin, scars, grafts and flaps
and factors which affect their condition*

*skin is the largest organ of the body, comprising approximately
16% of our weight; but sadly, it can be neglected and abused*

*we expect it to repair itself continually, to be healthy and look good,
to expand when necessary and to contract to its former size –
all without too much assistance from us…..*

a quick tour of skin, scars, grafts and flaps

It is important for you to understand the structure of skin, to be aware of different forms of scar tissue and the types of skin grafts and flaps used within reconstructive/plastic surgery.

Healthy skin is the body's first defence against the invasion of harmful bacteria, chemicals and foreign objects; it also helps to protect us from UV radiation.   It is a living, moist organ that has a visible dead surface, which naturally desquamates. It constantly renews itself although this process slows down with age. On average, it takes 28 days at the age of 20, gradually increasing to 37 days by the time we are 60-plus. Renewal is quicker where there is a hyperkeratinisation disorder, such as psoriasis.

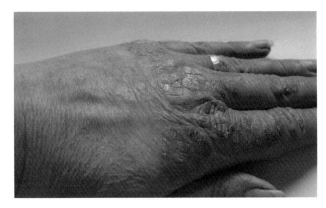
psoriasis

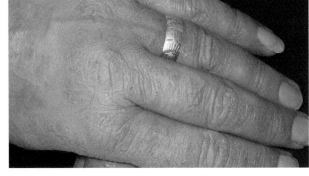
with camouflage application

Skin varies in thickness and texture, and is slightly thicker on men than on women. Where it is exposed to pressure (for example, on the palms and soles) it is thickest and hardest. Skin constantly exposed to UV becomes thicker

Skin has three layers,

- Epidermis (the outer layer)
- Dermis (the central layer)
- Subcutaneous (the deepest layer)

epidermis

as the epidermal cells (keratinocytes) migrate up through the epidermis to the outer, visible layer – the stratum corneum – they flatten, lose their nucleii, retain less moisture, become almost transparent and die. Consequently, the **corneum** is often referred to as the 'horny layer' because it is made up of cornified squames. The epidermis varies between 0.1mm and 1.4mm thick.

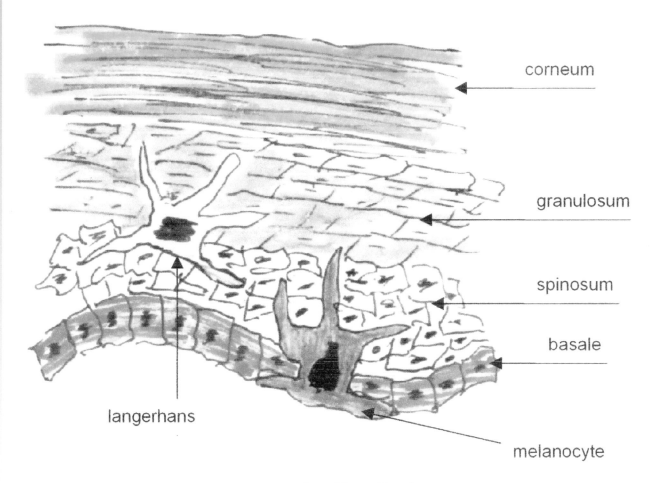

cross-section of the epidermis

In normal healthy skin the corneum has approximately 18 to 23 layers. It takes approximately 14 days for cells to migrate up the corneum before desquamation. Every day, approximately 4% of our total number of skin cells are shed from the corneum which, during a normal lifetime, adds about 13.5kg (30lbs) to household dust!

The underlying layers renew and replace the corneum. In ascending order the epidermal layers are:

stratum basale (basal layer): a single layer of cells where mitosis (the process of cell division) takes place every 200 to 400 hours

stratum spinosum: the upper part of the basal layer where most of the langerhans cells (which are responsible for the skin's immunological properties) are found. Production of keratin begins in this layer

stratum granulosum: where the cells begin to lose fluids and flatten

Skin cells float in a watery fluid that is slightly saline. Everyone is made up of 70% water, of which 35% is found in the skin. The basal layer contains approximately 80% water, with each subsequent layer holding less – the corneum being about 10–15%. It takes about 14 days for basal cells to migrate upwards before joining the base of the corneum. Another layer – the **stratum lucidum** – is considered to be a basement membrane which separates the corneum from the granulosum.

New cells produced in the basal layer contain pigment-forming melanocytes. We all have the same quantity of melanocytes, but the colour of our skin depends on our genetic predisposition and lifestyle.

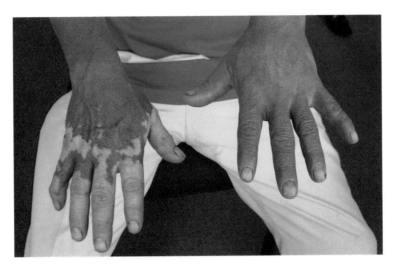

vitiligo to hands, his left hand only has camouflage applied
© BASC Member 2160 (at Aniquem, Peru)

In 1975, Thomas B Fitzpatrick MD PhD of Harvard Medical School, USA, developed a classification system based on the skin's response to sun exposure measured by the degree of burning and tanning experienced:

1 Highly sensitive to sun: always burns quickly, never achieves a tan
typically has very fair skin – tends to have multiple freckles, blue or green eyes, and auburn, blonde (but sometimes brunette) hair colouring

2 Very sun sensitive: burns easily, sometimes achieves a minimal tan
typically has fair skin, blue or brown eyes, fair to medium brunette hair

3 Sun sensitive: slowly tans to a light brown but burns with long exposure to sun
typically has medium skin colour, brown eyes and brunette to black hair

4 Minimally sensitive: tans to a moderate brown but can burn if skin exposed for very long periods to the sun
typically has light brown skin, brown eyes, dark brunette to black hair

5 Sun insensitive: tans well but can burn with excessive exposure to the sun
typically has medium brown skin, dark brown eyes, black hair

6 Sun insensitive : skin is naturally deeply pigmented and darkens easily, will only burn with extreme exposure to the sun
typically has very brown skin, black-brown eyes, black hair

**damage to the epidermis is superficial and quick to heal
and does not, normally, leave any permanent scarring
damaged melanocytes will permanently change the colour of the skin affected**

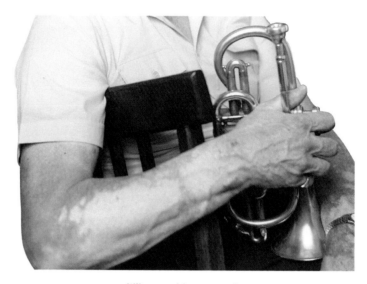

vitiligo – skin group 2
© the Vitiligo Association

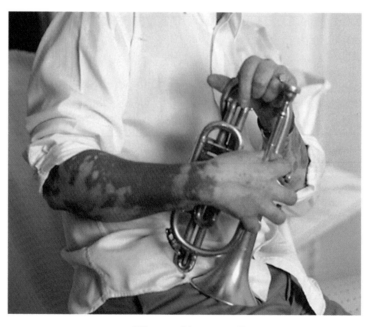

vitiligo – skin group 5
© the Vitiligo Association

pH value to the Acid Mantle of the Epidermis

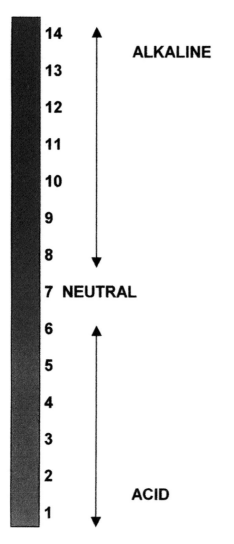

14
13
12
11
10
9
8
7 NEUTRAL
6
5
4
3
2
1

ALKALINE

ACID

The surface of healthy skin supports a mixture of resident bacteria and organic acids which is known as the 'acid mantle'. The acid mantle can be measured and given a pH value. The organic acids (produced by the keratinocytes) along with natural moisture and sebum form a secretion that helps to cement the cells together to prevent water loss and lowers the pH of the skin's surface to below 7. The resident bacteria are adapted to survive in this microenvironment without causing disease, and together with the low pH prevent colonisation by more harmful bacteria. It is important to maintain the pH balance for the skin to function properly as a barrier against microbial attack. There will be natural fluctuations due to resting, physical activity, type and amount of food and fluid intake, and cleansing of the skin. Such temporary change to the internal or external pH factor is a normal process and the acid mantle is quick to restore itself. Some skin conditions may slightly alter the acidity; a 'waxen' sheen to the skin may indicate a pH of 6.5+ which can be caused by any one of a number of medical conditions. It is important that medical attention is sought for an accurate diagnosis and treatment as cosmetic applications alone will not resolve the problem.

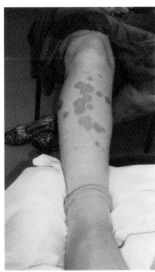

necrobiosis lipoidica
(condition associated with diabetes)
© BASC Member 1022

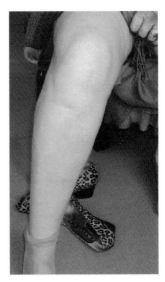

following skin camouflage application
© BASC Member 1022

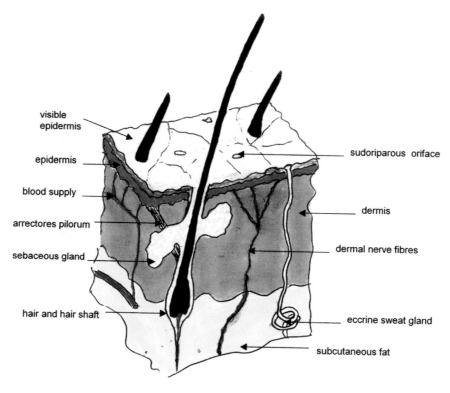

visible epidermis

epidermis

blood supply

arrectores pilorum

sebaceous gland

hair and hair shaft

sudoriparous oriface

dermis

dermal nerve fibres

eccrine sweat gland

subcutaneous fat

cross-section of skin

dermis

is thicker and stronger than the epidermis to which it supports. The dermis is a fibrous mass of tissue that includes elastin and collagen held in colloidal gel. It has an undulating form, which gradually loses elasticity with age and lifestyle leaving depressions, folds and dips (commonly referred to as wrinkles). The dermis varies between 0.6mm and 3mm thick.

The dermis contains capillaries, which supply blood to nourish the basal layer, sensory nerve endings, lymphocytes (cells that play an important part in the production of antibodies) and mast cells that release histamine

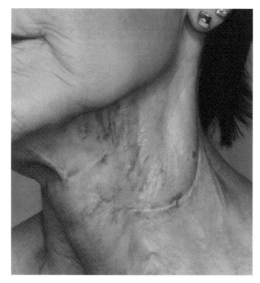

atrophic scarring and vascular malformation
© BASC Member 1022

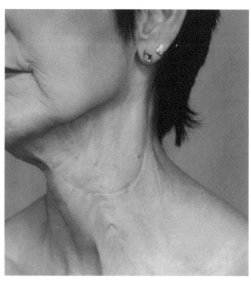

with skin camouflage applied
© BASC Member 1022

112

skin's defence mechanism

skin has always been considered waterproof, which suggests a one-way system for the outward passage of fluids that are designed to prevent the body from excessive loss of moisture. However, if the water loss is sufficient to destroy some of the living dermal cells as, for example, in the case of friction, burns and sunburn, then the mast cells are activated to release histamine. The visual sign is that the area becomes red because histamine dilates blood vessels. A blister containing serum is formed to protect the area from infection while the skin repairs itself. In urticaria (hives or nettle rash) histamine is released into the skin causing itchy red wheals to form.

The dermis renews itself at a slower rate than the epidermis: this means that damage to the dermis will take longer to heal. The dermis is referred to as connective tissue because it connects with the epidermis above and the subcutaneous below.

**damage to the dermis and subcutaneous layer will result in long-term
visual and physical alteration to the affected epidermis**

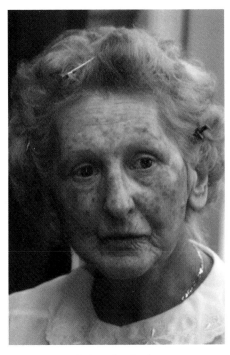

telangiectasia
© *Reynaud's and Scleroderma Association*

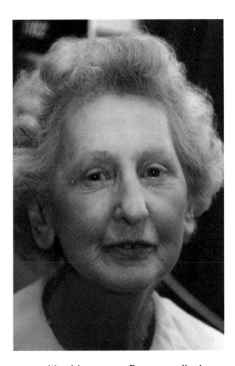

with skin camouflage applied
© *Reynaud's and Scleroderma Association*

subcutaneous

this layer has a network of lymphatic vessels that are interwoven with blood vessels and sensory nerves. It is also referred to as the adipose layer because it contains fat deposits, which act as a buffer to protect the underlying structure of the body and as an insulator against heat and cold. The fat helps to provide the body with contour. The thickness of subcutaneous tissue differs from one person to another and also varies from one area of the body to another.

sebaceous gland, hair and follicle

the epidermis inserts down into the dermis and subcutaneous tissue to create hair follicles. The longer the hair, the deeper the follicle will be. Each follicle has an appendage which contains one or more sebaceous glands that secrete sebum. Sebum is discharged through the pilosebaceous orifice: this helps to keep skin and hair supple and waterproof, and forms part of the corneum cement and pH value. Sebum also appears to have mild anti-bacterial and anti-fungal properties. Not every follicle will contain hair, or hair that is visible on the surface of the skin; some may contain multiple hairs. However, empty follicles continue to discharge sebum. This is especially so on the forehead, nose, above the upper lip and chin (sometimes referred to as the "T" zone).

Areas of the skin that do not contain hair follicles and sebaceous glands are the lips, palms, soles, nipples and certain parts of the sex organs.

Natural hair colour is controlled by melanocytes and whether it is straight or curled, fine or thick, quantity and distribution are all genetically predisposed.

Attached to each follicle is an arrectores pilorum muscle. This contracts and makes the hair stand erect in response to fright or cold, and gives the skin an uneven texture commonly known as 'goose pimples'.

The body has two types of hair: the fine, downy vellus hair that coats most of the skin, and the coarser terminal hair on the scalp, eyelashes and eyebrows. During hormonal changes at puberty some of the vellus hair follicles alter to produce coarser terminal hair: these are in the groin, in the axillae and on men to form beard growth.

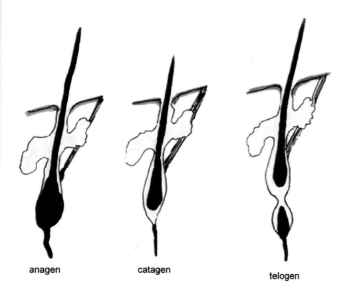

anagen   catagen   telogen

hair growth cycle

Hair growth has three stages:
- anagen: the growing stage
- catagen: growth stops and the papilla begins to retract
- telogen: the hair becomes detached from the follicle and eventually falls away, when the follicle rests until anagen starts again.

Humans have a randomised hair growth-shedding pattern with the timescale differing between sites. For example, eyebrow hairs grow faster but last approximately four months, whereas scalp hair anagen can be for 3 to 7 years before telogen (we normally shed 50-100 scalp hairs every 24 hours).

It is generally thought that hair quantity reduction using IPL and suitable LASER equipment is best achieved when the hair is at anagen. On the whole, the darker the hair colour, and the more pale the skin colour, the better the outcome. At the time of going to print there is no effective IPL or LASER to remove blonde and grey hair.

**excessive sebum production will adversely affect
the durability-stability of skin camouflage
crème camouflage does not adhere to hair (excluding scalp hair)**

sudoriparous (sweat) glands

sweat glands have ducts that coil up through the dermis and epidermis to deposit water containing waste material onto the skin's surface. There are two types of sweat gland: eccrine and apocrine.

eccrine glands control the body's temperature by flooding the external layer of the corneum to cool the skin. There are eccrine glands throughout the skin but they are most numerous on the palms and soles. Most of the sweat evaporates, but some remains within the corneum to help hydration. A typical insensitive perspiration rate is approximately 0.5 litre every 24 hours.

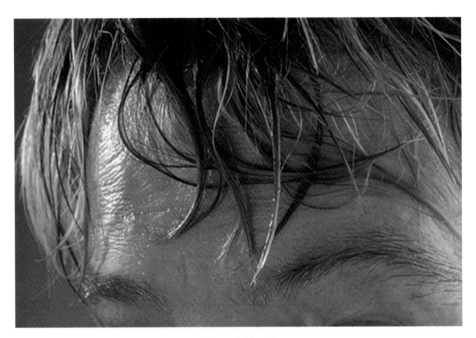

Hyperhidrosis
© Hyperhidrosis Support Group

apocrine glands are activated by hormones during and just after puberty. They do not contribute to, nor are they controlled by, the body's temperature mechanism. Apocrine sweat is a granular, milky secretion containing pheromone which forms part of the social-sexual scent signals. Unfortunately apocrine sweat also attracts bacteria which, in turn, produces the unpleasant smell commonly known as body odour.

hyperhidrosis will adversely affect the durability-stability of skin camouflage

scars

a scar indicates a healed wound – it is produced as a result of the body's normal healing mechanism when skin has been damaged. If the damage has affected all the skin's layers, or has taken a long time to heal, the scar will take longer to mature. Mature scar tissue, which may have a smooth or puckered edge, can be broadly categorised as being one of the following:

atrophic (indented): also referred to as normal scar tissue: the scar is stretched and the dermis thinned

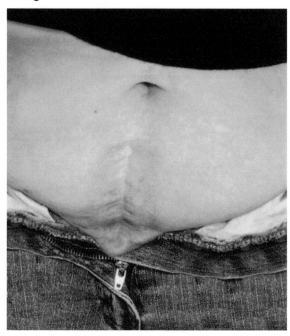

01 *mature atrophic*

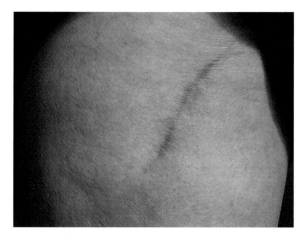

03 *normal scarring, one year old*

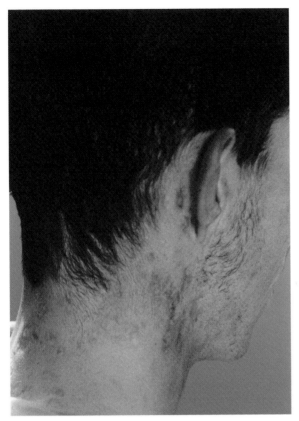

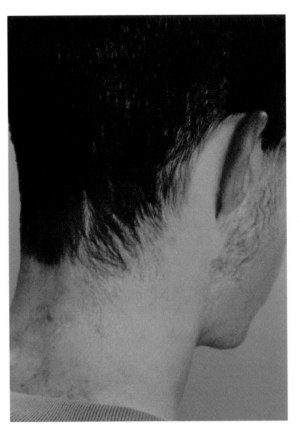

01 post acne "ice pick" scarring

01 camouflage result

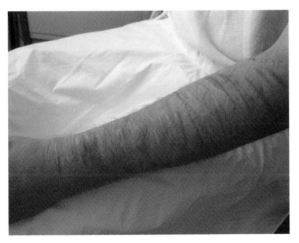

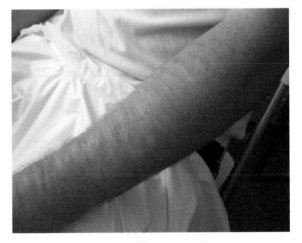

hypertrophic scarring
© BASC Member 2303

camouflage result
© BASC Member 2303

hypertrophic (raised): excess collagen makes the scar protrude higher than the surrounding skin

keloid (nodular): excessive collagen creates undulating scar tissue that is very firm to the touch and extends over normal tissue.

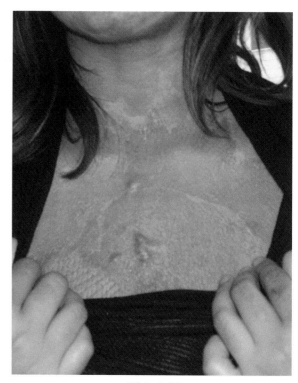

03 *keloid*

plastic surgery techniques

plastic surgery procedures are required when skin is extensively damaged and cannot repair itself. Plastic surgery was known about and practised for the treatment of burns in China 5,000 BC and Egypt 3,000 BC. In India (600BC) surgeons used skin from foreheads to reconstruct noses; Hippocrates (400 BC) also used reconstructive surgery techniques. The Roman doctor Cornelius Celsus is credited with the first writings about such operations in his De Medicina (AD30). Modern plastic surgery dates from around 1885 when local anaesthetics were invented. In 1887 John Roe of New York published The Deformity Termed Pug Nose. Howard Kelly of Baltimore performed the first removal of abdominal fat (15lbs) in 1889. Eugene Hollander (Berlin 1901) is credited for the first facelift; his patient was a Polish aristocrat who provided detailed sketches of what he wanted achieved. Historically, however, the real pioneers come from Great Britain; Sir Astley Cooper performed the first skin graft in humans (1817); other luminaries, such as Sir Harold Gillies and Sir Archibald McIndoe, belong to the 20th century *(for additional information see A Potted History of Skin Camouflage)*

skin grafts

is when skin is taken from a donor area and secured on the recipient area. The small capillaries then work into the tissue as it heals.   Skin grafts are classified as either split-thickness or full-thickness grafts,

- split-thickness grafts consist of the epidermis and a portion of the dermis; may also be called a spilt skin graft and abbreviated as SSG
- full-thickness grafts include the entire thickness of epidermis and dermis; may also be called a Wolfe Graft and abbreviated as FTWG (full thickness Wolfe graft)

The advantages and disadvantages of split-thickness and full-thickness grafts are,

split-thickness
a split-thickness graft is versatile in the areas it can cover provided the bed on which it is to be placed has a good blood supply.

advantages
can take under less favourable conditions; can cover large areas

disadvantages
can shrink considerably; unpredictable pigmentation; highly susceptible to trauma

The SSG can be used in two ways,
- to take a sufficient quantity to cover the defect and lay over the area as "a sheet graft"
- to extend the area of coverage and create a mesh graft; which is achieved by placing the skin through a meshing machine for perforation which will allow the skin to stretch and extend.

sheet skin graft
has the advantage that it will heal more quickly and give a better cosmetic outcome. The disadvantage is that there is a smaller area of coverage which can be more at risk by collections of blood or serous fluid under the graft reducing the "take".

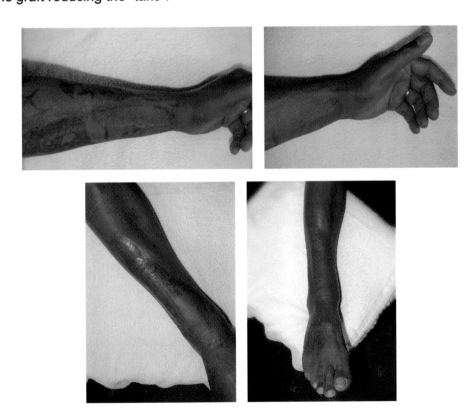

partial tattoo from the donor site on the arm has transferred with the graft to the leg 04

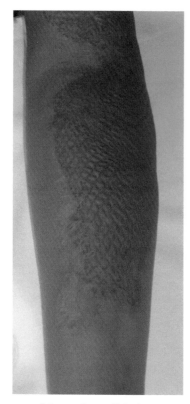
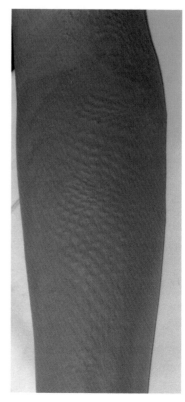

03 mesh graft before   *03 with skin camouflage*

mesh skin graft

can cover a greater area and conforms well to awkward areas, such as elbows and knees. The perforations allow the blood and serous fluid to escape. However mesh grafts give a poor cosmetic result and take longer to heal as the gaps over the exposed dermis needs to re-epithelise

full-thickness

a full thickness graft is always a sheet graft

advantages

contracts much less than a SSG; has the potential for growth; the texture and pigment is more similar to normal skin

disadvantages

will require a well-vascularised bed

flaps

differ from skin grafts in that it contains structures such as muscle, bone, nerves, and fascia, with or without the skin. A flap is raised with its own blood supply then plumbed in to the recipient area

A flap is used to cover areas without an adequate base layer where bulk is required to fill a cavity or where other structures are needed to maintain form and / or function. Flaps are commonly used to reconstruct,

-   the breast following mastectomy
-   areas where large tumours have been removed
-   post trauma where there is extensive loss of tissue

Flaps are classified in various ways,

according to their composition
-   cutaneous - skin only
-   fasciocutaneous - fascia and skin
-   myocutaneous - muscle and skin
-   osseomyocutaneous - bone, muscle and skin
-   innervated (sensate) cutaneous - nerve and skin

according to their blood supply
-   random flaps, supplied by one or more arteries where their inclusion in the flap base occurs by random selection
-   axial flaps, supplied by named arteries that run longitudinally along the axis of the flap

according to the method of movement.
-   local transfer : advancement, rotation, transposition
-   distant transfer : direct, tubed, microvascular free

tissue expansion

is a technique that relies on the principle that skin grows when slowly stretched from underneath. Think about pregnancy and how the skin grows.

A balloon device is inserted under the skin in an area near the scar. The device is filled by injecting saline into it in small amounts over a period of time. When there is sufficient skin the device is removed and the excess skin used to cover the defect.

This is a useful technique when there is scarring on the scalp and hair-bearing skin is needed to cover. However, it thins out the follicles and can only cover small areas. It is also used sometimes to remove very clumped up scars.

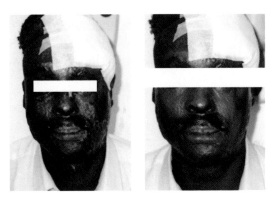

tissue expansion in progress (camouflage applied to facial hypo pigmentation)
© BASC Member 1022

121

factors which affect the condition of skin and scars

although only the uppermost layer of the corneum is visible, we can classify 'skin' into four hereditary types and four categories that are affected by internal and external factors.

Recognising the person's complexion (type and category) will help you select the camouflage product that will best suit their skin.

hereditary skin types are:
- normal
- oily
- dry
- combination

with their condition being potentially affected and categorised as:
- dehydrated
- mature
- sensitive
- sun-damaged.

Most skins will combine more than one type and one category. For example, a dry skin may also be mature and sun-damaged, or an oily skin can be dehydrated on the cheeks but generally sensitive to some cosmetic ingredients.

normal

before puberty a healthy child could be said to have a 'normal' skin – this means there is sufficient sebum to prevent any signs of dryness but not too much to cause a greasy shine. At this stage of development the skin also contains the necessary water to keep it fine, smooth, evenly textured and soft. However, changes occur during and after puberty. A face with 'normal' skin is usually the luxury of the young! Puberty, lifestyle, the environment, genetic background and the ageing process all contribute to make skin less than this balanced complexion.

oily

although problematic, oily skin usually can have the benefit of not showing the signs of ageing as quickly as other skin types. Oily skin shines but can also look 'cloudy' because too much sebum glues the squames on the surface and prevents normal desquamation. This can block the sweat pores and hair follicles, which will create comedo (comedones, blackheads, a plug of keratin and sebum in the orifice of a sebaceous gland) and milium (milia, tiny white cysts of keratin). The larger the sebaceous gland, the bigger the pilosebaceous orifice will need to be to accommodate it and to discharge sebum. This is often described as 'having large pores', which cosmetic manufacturers claim can be minimised with use of a topical product. Unfortunately, any 'shrinking of pores' is extremely temporary. If you have large sebaceous glands and, by definition, large follicles you will always have, and need, 'large pores'. Increased hormonal activity during puberty can cause an imbalance of glandular secretions. This might lead to an over-production of sebum by the sebaceous glands, which can lead to conditions such as seborrhoea and acne.

dry

although the skin appears flaky and is prone to small cracks, the water content of dry skin is the same as that of normal skin. Dry skin has under-active sebaceous glands, resulting in insufficient sebum secretion to prevent water loss. The skin looks delicate and thin because there is insufficient cellular cement to bond the horny layers together. As it does not always fully desquamate, the skin feels rough to the touch, is often itchy and has a dull, matt appearance. Dermatosis, such as psoriasis and scleroderma, can create very dry lesions.

combination

after puberty everyone could be classified as having a 'combination skin'. A 'T' shape is used to describe the areas of the forehead, nose, upper lip and chin where there is a natural abundance of sebum secretion. Combination skin is typically described as having a shine to the 'T' area (with the potential for comedones) and less so on the cheeks where it may be dry. However, a combination skin can be sensitive and normal or, indeed, any combination of the conditions and categories. When applying cosmetics and toiletries, the differing areas may need appropriate products.

dehydrated

can affect all skin types, although it is most often associated and confused with dry skin. It is caused by an excessive loss of water from the skin, aggravated by cold, sun, central heating, wind, air conditioning, over-use of astringents and frequent cleansing with soap and water. Excessive sweating also increases dehydration. Dehydrated dry skin has the characteristics of dry skin and can easily become chapped, itchy, sore and red. Dehydrated oily skin causes the oil secretion to block pores and trap sebum within the corneum, which will adversely affect skin prone to comedones or acne.

mature

as skin matures, its renewal process begins to slow down, as does the production of sebum. With less sebum, the capacity to retain water decreases and this makes the skin more vulnerable to dehydration. Menopausal women may find the changes in their skin sudden and dramatic – the reduction of hormones in men causes a more gradual change as male skin ages at a slower rate than female. As we age the skin becomes drier and thinner. It can be easily damaged by the slightest bump or knock.

sensitive

all skin types and conditions may experience sensitivity when an allergy reaction is triggered. The cause of the allergy is individual and not necessarily associated with a cosmetic application. For example, although someone's forehead may show classic primary irritant symptoms, the allergy may be caused by an ingredient in a shampoo rather than by a topical crème or decorative cosmetic.

sun-damaged

a suntan is the visual symptom of skin protecting you against ultraviolet (UV) damage. UV radiation (either by natural sun or from solariums and sun lamps) causes solar lentigo, telangiectasia, fine lines and wrinkles, and irregular pigmentation. Exposure increases the long-term risk of skin cancers and of cataract formation in the lens of the eye.

UVA is mostly absorbed in the epidermis but can penetrate the dermis where it causes photoageing by damaging the elasticity of the skin. Sunbeds and sunlamps emit UVA.

UVB causes erythema and sunburn to the epidermis and will also stimulate thickening of the corneum. UVB triggers essential vitamin D synthesis.

When exposed to the sun, skin will defend itself by producing extra melanin. People who have prolonged exposure to the sun (whether due to working or playing outdoors) will also develop thicker, but far less supple, yellowed skin – even when using sunscreens.

UV phototherapy and photochemotherapy can be used to treat certain conditions. However, dermatoses can react differently to sun exposure (some with psoriasis may show an improvement whereas the sun may be the a trigger for others) and vitiligo patches will quickly sunburn, even on a cloudy day.

Skin can, and does, recover if moderately exposed to sun, but to minimise the harmful effects of ultraviolet, children and adults must be educated to frequently apply a product that protects them from UVA and UVB.

scars

the sun is also a great enemy to scars. Avoidance is the preferred option, or use of a total sunblock of at least factor 30. All scars (as well as some dermatosis) will be more fragile and sensitive and care must be taken when using perfumes, soaps and clothing containing synthetic fibres.

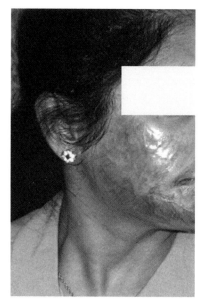

scarring from a burn injury
© BASC Member 1022

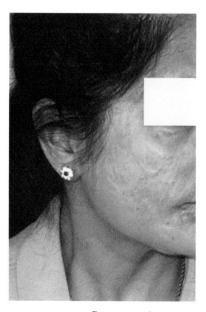

camouflage result
© BASC Member 1022

A scar (whether it is atrophic, hypertrophic or keloid) will usually be dry and may feel different to the surrounding skin. This is because when the skin heals, hair follicles (with their attached sebaceous glands) and sweat glands are interrupted, which changes the pH to the scar. The need for emollients may continue indefinitely to keep the skin supple and prevent dehydration, cracking or splitting. Scars do benefit from gentle massage as this also helps to keep the skin hydrated.

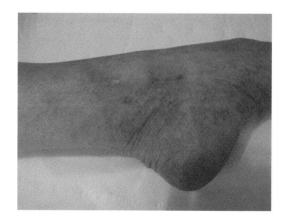

pigmented scar from healed ulcer
© BASC Member 2249
The British Association of Sclerotherapy

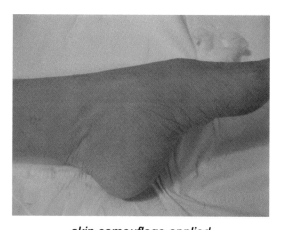

skin camouflage applied
© BASC Member 2249
The British Association of Sclerotherapy

After a wound is healed the scar will form normally, but in some cases it may become red and slightly raised and develop into hypertrophic scarring. With proper management (using pressure dressings and/ or silicone treatments) the hypertrophy will eventually settle down, this can take up to 6 to 12 months. Given time scars usually improve, but this whole process may take 12 to 24 months. Irrespective of maturity, scars can continue to itch and be painful or tender to the lightest pressure.

Major keloid scars can continue to increase in size over several years and can develop many years after the initial injury. Keloid scars occur more often on skin groups 4 to 6 (the reasons for this are unknown) and may result from the simplest of injuries, such as a bee sting. There have been reports of skin groups 1 to 3 developing keloid tissue, which appears to be a direct result of body piercing and wearing several rings in one area (especially ears). Anyone predisposed to keloid scars should be advised not to have any tattoos or piercing.

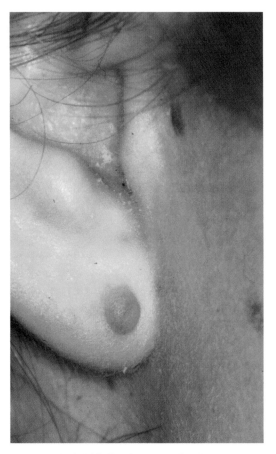

keloid following ear piercing

**camouflage products are designed to disguise a predominant colour and
to match in and blend with the natural colour of the surrounding skin
sadly they cannot return a scar or dermatosis to align with the natural skin**

an overview of psychology and the conditions most frequently referred for skin camouflage

what may seem to be a small and insignificant mark to the camouflage practitioner can assume enormous proportions and implications for the patient

an overview of psychology and the conditions most frequently referred for skin camouflage

This chapter gives a brief overview of the conditions most frequently referred for skin camouflage, together with their special considerations. Unless suggested otherwise, all skin matching and camouflage application follows usual practice.

There are over 2,000 known diseases of the skin, most of which are less than common and can be considered rare. It is therefore impractical for camouflage practitioners to be familiar with all dermatoses. However, depending on the needs of your workplace, it will be useful for you to make a more specialist study than this book allows. There are excellent books on dermatology and skin disorders that can be used as a reference guide to different medical conditions and most have photographs, which is particularly useful before meeting anyone with a dermatosis that you have not seen before. The British Association of Dermatologists has excellent Patient Information Leaflets that can be downloaded from their website, as too do Patient Support Groups directly.

We advise caution when camouflage is requested for children. The camouflage practitioner will need to distinguish (carefully and tactfully) who is requesting the consultation and why - is it the child or the family, and for what purpose? We appreciate that most prepubescent children do not seek skin camouflage; however, it may be that the camouflage practitioner has not been made aware of the reasons why the medical advisor and/or psychologist recommends camouflage at an earlier age. Camouflage is not rub proof, and children are very tactile! This may mean that greater psychological problems are caused with transfer of product onto another, or onto toys, or school equipment. It is good practice to direct people to Patient Support Groups who have the specialist skills to advise adults and support children who have a visible difference.

Unfortunately this chapter allows only for an overview on the psychology and recommended language to use during your skin camouflage service. We strongly suggest that you do not counsel anyone unless you are a qualified to do so and as part of a multi-disciplinary team you might suggest the person seeks colleague's specialist advice.

Always remember that someone has come to you for skin camouflage advice and keep within the boundary of your qualifications.

language can become a barrier, rather than an aid to understanding

jargon

your colleagues will be familiar with your specialism's terminology – but is your jargon a handicap to widespread communication? Not everyone will immediately understand a "lesion" (to indicate a section, area or patch) "presenting" (being visible) on their skin and requiring a "topical" (applied to the corneum) "preparation" (lotion, potion or medication) to be used.

People do not always remember the medical name of their skin condition, some of which are difficult to say and to spell. This is especially so when people receive a lot of information in a short space of time. Most do not want to cause embarrassment by asking you for simple explanations and will just "nod" that they understand.

It is vital that you use language which is easy for people to understand and make certain that the person requesting camouflage follows your advice. Consideration must also be given to people whose main language is not English and for those who cannot read English. In order to address any problems in translation, we created a pictorial reminder of how to apply camouflage. It was a bonus to learn that this is also very useful when explaining camouflage routines to children.

In order for people to identify with and adjust to a change in their image all language used needs to include them, and not be exclusive. BASC have long campaigned for caution with the following negative terminology:

failure

people who are struggling to adjust to their altered image may be feeling uncertain about their future (as defined in the Stages of Grief – see overleaf). This may affect their education, their domestic and social life and employment. People often use the word "failure" to describe their feelings of anxiety. Unfortunately the phrase "failed to attend" is frequently recorded by professionals on people's medical notes and used within correspondence to those who, for whatever personal reason, did not attend the consultation. There will be a variety of reasons why someone has missed an appointment - the use of "failed to attend" can only contribute and endorse someone's insecurities and feelings of failure.

disabled.

when we asked people if they considered themselves disabled by their skin condition and scarring, the majority did not identify themselves with this description. People with burn injury contracture, psoriatic arthritis and those whose skin condition causes loss of mobility, hearing or sight considered themselves to be less able than before; but there was a general reluctance to accept the label of "disabled". The majority thought it might encourage misunderstanding and negativity to their skin condition.

disfigured

our questioning highlighted that people only identified with this label following severe facial trauma that resulted in them wearing prosthesis, such as an artificial eye, prosthetic nose or ear. Most agreed (including those with skin grafts) that their skin condition caused them inconveniences and loss of self-esteem, but they did not identify at all with being "disfigured".

Although our informal survey should not be considered conclusive evidence, it did confirm that language can be destructive as well as constructive.

We recommend you do not use the above failure – disabled – disfigured labels, especially when talking to, or about children, vulnerable teenagers and young adults because these terms are so powerful they may be the "tipping point" for someone to develop other behaviours, such as eating disorders or self harm.

Language is so powerful
that we need to look at how it is used
when talking about disfigurement.
Here at the Centre we talk of 'visible difference'
which is a neutral term I would like to see used by everyone".

Professor Nichola Rumsey
Centre for Appearance Research (Bristol)
Daily Telegraph 15th December 2014

emotional adjustment for an altered image

Psychologists consider that we experience the same emotional stages to a change to our image as those experienced during bereavement.

It is might be more accurate to term these as "components" rather than stages because they do not necessarily follow in any given order. However, only when the first seven have been successfully worked through can Resolution be reached. Although Ramsey and de Groot[1] identified nine components, Shock and Disorganisation, and Resolution and Re-Integration are often grouped together.

Each component may last from a few moments to several weeks, months or even years (the timeframe being individual) and some people may never fully attain resolution and re-integration.

1. **SHOCK**
2. **DISORGANISATION**
3. **DENIAL**
4. **DEPRESSION**
5. **GUILT**
6. **ANXIETY**
7. **AGGRESSION**
8. **RESOLUTION**
9. **RE-INTEGRATION**

In relation to an altered image, the suggested overview of the person's emotional condition is:

SHOCK
a feeling of astonishment and disbelief this has happened

DISORGANISATION
thoughts are preoccupied, making it difficult to achieve the simplest things

DENIAL
behaves as if nothing has happened, unwilling to comply to treatment

DEPRESSION
despair and powerlessness that anything can rectify the situation

GUILT
neglect (real or imagined) of being responsible for what has happened

ANXIETY
apprehension about the future (work, social and financial)

AGGRESSION
irritability or anger to self and others as to why this has happened

RESOLUTION
acceptance emerges, willingness to comply to treatments

RE-INTEGRATION
return to acceptable lifestyle

Skin camouflage may be rejected and not be considered an option until the person nears Resolution, but it may be of some comfort for them to know skin camouflage can help - it is something they may wish to explore later in their rehabilitation. Some may consider that their need for skin camouflage diminishes over time and perhaps disappears altogether. For others there is the choice to use skin camouflage at a frequency that suits their need.

---

[1] Cited by P E Hodgkinson in The Nursing Times 17.01.1980 (p126-128) *Treating Abnormal Grief in the Bereaved.* Also see *Psychology, The Science of Mind & Behavior* by Richard Gross; *The Nine Components of Grief* by R Ramsay and W de Groot, 1977 – taken from paper presented at European Addiction Training Institute Conference, Uppsala University, Stockholm, Sweden, *A Further Look At Bereavement.*

conditions most frequently referred for skin camouflage

acne
this affects the pilosebaceous gland and involves four inter-related factors,

- increased levels of circulating androgens during puberty lead to a surge in sebum production, causing oily skin
- the cells lining the pilosebaceous follicles become sticky and clump together; this blocks the orifice, allowing the sebum to pool
- the oil then solidifies and becomes pigmented, leading to comedones and milia
- due to abnormal function of the ductal bacteria Proprioni bacterium (P.acnes) colonises, which causes inflammation

clinical features
acne predominantly affects the face, neck, chest and back. It presents as comedones, papules, nodules, cysts and scars. If no comedones are present then it is not acne. It is easily recognised as,

Mild	comedones with few inflamed lesions
Moderate	many inflamed lesions, with pustules also present (scarring may also be present)
Severe	extensive nodules, cysts and scarring, normally affecting all sites

special considerations
the psychological impact of acne is often severely under-estimated. It is a very visible condition that can cause permanent scarring. It can cause young people to isolate themselves at a time when relationships are an important part of their psychological development. Acne is not only confined to teenagers and can affect people into their 40s and 50s. It can have major socio-economic implications with career options potentially reduced.

dispelling social myths
despite a large amount of research, there is no evidence to support the notion that acne is caused by eating chips, fried foods, chocolate and so on. It is not caused by bad hygiene or not washing. Acne is not contagious. Covering it up with make-up (and skin camouflage) should not make it worse. It is important for people to wear make-up if they want to, but cosmetic products should be non-comedogenic. Some acne medications can increase sensitivity to sunlight, so it is important that a non-comedogenic sunscreen is used.

acne ('ice pick' scarring)
predisposition is mild but severe forms of acne (see above) when large nodules and cysts distort the follicle, rupture into the surrounding dermis and create scarring.

clinical features
atrophic pitting of the skin (often described as 'ice pick' scarring). Hypertrophic and keloid scars occur most often on the chest and back of young adults with severe acne.

dispelling social myths
acne does not only affect young men – women are equally affected – and both are affected by the social stigma associated with a scarred face.

camouflage for acne and acne scarring
camouflage can be used to good effect to help conceal acne scarring but must be discontinued immediately following dermabrasion/chemical peels until the medical advisor gives permission for the person to continue their application.

Camouflage products, because they are generally non-comedogenic, are ideal, especially to conceal erythema and hyperpigmentation. However, some people may prefer to use oil-free (powder) camouflage, but there is no evidence to support that oil-based camouflage encourages acne.

capillary and superficial cavernous haemangiomas

a benign, raised and distorted area, which can develop quickly after birth or during the first few months of life. The can also be referred to as "strawberry birth marks", "stork kisses" and "salmon patches".

clinical features
They are usually found on the face but can appear on the limbs or trunk. Capillary haemangiomas are bright pink or red areas; cavernous are similar but deeper and bluish in colour.

dispelling social myths
There is no truth whatsoever that the cause was the mother eating strawberries, or other red fruits or vegetables, or salmon during pregnancy. Neither is it true that the stork kissed the baby on delivery!

camouflage
Given the age of the child, it is usually totally inappropriate to apply skin camouflage. However, if the family requests camouflage for a special occasion when photographs will be taken, then it may be appropriate to consider camouflage for that event only. The camouflage practitioner will need to distinguish carefully to see who is requesting camouflage and why – is it the child or the family and for what purpose?

chloasma/melasma

chloasma (also known as melasma) is dependent on exposure to sunlight combined with a hormone imbalance, and believed to be triggered by UV rays reacting with oestrogen to produce lesions of excess melanin production. It usually affects women, but can also affect men, and seems to be more common in skin groups 2-4. Triggers can include pregnancy (and is often regarded as "the mask of pregnancy") and taking oral contraceptive pills and hormone replacement therapy (HRT) which contain oestrogen. It is also thought that topical applications, especially perfumed products or hormonal cremes, may activate this condition. There is no know cure.

clinical features
hyperpigmented lesions on face and neck, usually around the eyes, on the cheeks, forehead and upper lip.

dispelling social myths
although associated with taking the oral contraceptive pill or HRT, the condition also occurs in women who have no known hormonal imbalance and are not taking any oestrogen-based medication. It also occurs in women who are not pregnant, or have never been.

camouflage
there is usually a blue undertone to the lesion. Try a complementary pale rose red (skin group 1), pale terracotta (for skin groups 2 to 3), terracotta (for skin groups 4 to -5), deep red rose (skin group 6) under the skin match.

cleft lip

despite cleft lip and palate being the most common anomaly of the head and neck, the causes are not fully understood. It does tend to run in families, but also occurs in isolation.

clinical features

someone born with a cleft lip may have a visible scar running between the nose and the mouth. Their nose may also have a slightly irregular shape. Someone born with a cleft palate may have irregular teeth and a slightly unusual jaw line. Some syndromes, which feature cleft palate, might also affect the appearance (such as Pierre Robin syndrome, which features a small lower jaw). People may lack confidence as a result of looking and/or sounding different to other people.

dispelling social myths

cleft lip and palate have been associated in the past with undesirable qualities in people, and the condition has been used in literature to indicate an undesirable or flawed character. Cleft lip and palate is also sometimes wrongly associated with lesser developmental and/or learning abilities. Though some syndromes featuring cleft palate might be connected with learning difficulties, cleft lip and/or palate alone is not. These unacceptable attitudes might still have an influence on people's perception of the condition today.

camouflage

if the scar tissue distorts the lip shape, camouflage, lip stains or medical tattooing can be used to redefine the lip.

congenital melanocytic naevi and moles

cause unknown, usually hereditary. More common in skin groups 1 to 3. A naevus is a collection of melanocytic cells; they are usually benign and can be visible at birth but generally develop as the child grows up and into adulthood. Congenital melanocytic naevi (CMN) present at birth, or develop soon afterwards.

clinical features

moles range from dark brown to black hyperpigmented spots, varying in size and number, in some instances raised and/or with hair growing. Congenital melanocytic naevi may also have lumpy areas. People must be made aware to check their moles for changes in colour, shape, size and to discontinue camouflage until medical opinion confirms the lesion is benign.

dispelling social myths

a single mole on the upper lip or side of the chin has, throughout history, been considered as a 'beauty spot' whereas a profusion of moles on the face or chest has been considered the markings of witchcraft.

camouflage

a yellow-white complementary may be needed for lighter brown naevi on skin groups 1 to 3. For black naevi, a pastel orange complementary on skin groups 1 to 3 and dark terracotta complementary to skin groups 4 to 6 will resolve any ghosting through.

discoid lupus erythematosus

is an autoimmune disorder, mainly affecting areas where skin is exposed to sun (particularly the face, neck and cape areas, upper trunk and hands) including the scalp, which may result in permanent hair loss. Discoid lupus usually only affects the skin, but some might develop systemic lupus (which causes excess antibodies in the blood stream causing inflammation and damage in the joints, muscles and other organs).

clinical features

the condition presents as symmetrical, well-defined areas of erythema, with scaling, atrophy and blocked hair follicles.

dispelling social myths

some people wrongly believe that the condition is infectious.

camouflage

scaling may present problems similar to psoriasis.

ephelides (freckles)

a freckle is due to spontaneous, localised increase in the production of melanin by a normal quota of melanocytes.

clinical features

multiple freckles mainly affect skin groups 1, usually on the face, cape and limbs. Freckles darken and proliferate with exposure to sunlight, and can merge to form large patches.

dispelling social myths

although Titian haired groups have a predisposition to freckles, people may wrongly believe that all redheads have freckles and associate this with being 'hot tempered'. Children can be taunted and this can lead to loss of self-image and behavioural problems.

camouflage

it is inappropriate to 'dot' camouflage freckle by freckle, therefore the whole area including normal pigmented skin should be covered.

Kaposi's sarcoma (KS)

may manifest when there is a breakdown of the immune system and is often seen in people with AIDS and those who misuse drugs. KS may also result from the neurological condition neurofibromatosis. It causes internal lesions in various places, such as the lymph nodes, lungs and intestines, and external lesions on the skin (face and body).

clinical features

lesions are not usually painful, can be various sizes and shapes, often raised, hard and sometimes shiny. They are red, reddish-brown, and dark-blue to purple in colour, which may resemble a bruise, a blood blister or a love bite.

dispelling social myths

KS can affect anyone: gay or straight, with or without AIDS. The lesions are not contagious. KS probably gives most concern because it is so recognisable and for some people, KS will represent an AIDS diagnosis. It is important to be aware that the person is also coming to terms with the traumatic implications of transition from HIV to AIDS, as well as coping with skin lesions. In some cases they may not have even been aware of being HIV positive. People are extremely vulnerable and may even be suicidal, so will require your patience, understanding, tact and empathy. People who develop KS because of other medical conditions can incorrectly be assumed to have AIDS.

camouflage

lesions can be dealt with in the normal way; a complementary may be required on very hyperpigmentated areas. In order to create a natural appearance to the camouflaged area, the best results can be achieved using a fixier spray to give a semi-shiny, rather than matt finish. This is particularly useful when camouflage is applied to the tip of the nose where KS is frequently found.

lentigines and solar lentigo

spontaneous, localised increase in melanocyte production but, unlike ephelides, the marks doe not increase or darken in colour when exposed to sunlight. The cause of solar lentigo is over-exposure to sunlight, lentigines can be evident in children but become more prevalent with age, when they are usually called 'liver spots' and 'age spots'.

clinical features

lentigines can be slightly raised, well distributed, large 'freckles' that are very dark brown to black coloured. Solar lentigo may be lighter in colour and have an irregular shape.

dispelling social myths

there is no clinical evidence that excessive drinking and eating causes liver spots.

camouflage

follow advice given for congenital melanocytic naevi.

naevus flammeus (port wine stain)

visible at birth, this is a developmental defect of dermal capillaries and is permanent. May affect the eye if it is in that vicinity, and can also affect underlying organs and need further investigation. The growth of an affected limb should be checked regularly by the appropriate specialist.

clinical features

present as dark pink to purple-red to dark-brown lesions that are usually confined to one side of the face, neck or body; the lesions can be pale at birth, or flat, but may develop into large and raised dark pigmented areas as the child gets older.

dispelling social myths

given that this capillary malformation occurs during the first trimester of pregnancy, many mothers feel guilty, quite wrongly, that it may have been something they ate or did wrong. Some folklore accuses the mother of not satisfying a food craving, while others accuse the mother of over-eating red coloured foods and drinking claret. Also totally untrue is the belief that the shape of the mark denotes its source: for example, resembling the numbers 666 has some devil influence or that a clover or horseshoe shape may cause the child to live a charmed life.

camouflage

a complementary colour is rarely needed.

neurofibromatosis (café au lait marks)

the cause is hereditary: marks may be present at birth or may develop later, but may have a neurological association.

clinical features

light brown (resembling milky coffee) splashes of hyperpigmented skin, which can vary in size from small to large. The quantity of marks will vary, and some may become dome shaped raised above the skin.

dispelling social myths

there is no clinical evidence to support the myth that the mother drank too much coffee or tea.

camouflage

follow the suggestions given for congenital melanocytic naevi.

psoriasis

a hereditary condition that is associated with autoimmune but may occur during times of hormonal change such as puberty, pregnancy and the menopause. It is often associated with temporary ill health and may follow trauma to the skin (Koebner phenomenon). It occurs in all races. There is no known cure once triggered but some may find spontaneous relief or temporary respite. In simple terms, the condition is caused by an over-production of skin (up to every four days) which results in layers of squames (plaques) accumulating on the surface.

There are many different types of psoriasis, not all suitable for camouflage including,

- erythrodermic psoriasis
- generalised pustular psoriasis
- persistent palmoplantar pustulosis

clinical features

plaque psoriasis

is the most common form and has well-defined borders of itchy, red plaques with characteristically silvery white scales, which when sloughed or scratched off may cause bleeding. It is usually sited on the knees, elbows and extensor surfaces but may also present elsewhere.

flexural psoriasis

the areas usually lose their scales and appear as bright, shiny red lesions.

guttate and exanthematic psoriasis:

present as multiple small lesions, usually on the limbs and trunk – more common in young people and may follow a throat infection. The condition may develop into plaque psoriasis or disappear spontaneously.

psoriatic arthropathy

this presents as arthritis to any joint and most commonly affects the toes, fingers and lower back. The arthritic sites may or may not have psoriasis plaques.

dispelling social myths

there is little evidence to suggest that the trigger for psoriasis is totally psychological. However, people who lead stressful lives may also be less vigilant with their diet and sleep patterns which, in turn, could contribute to triggering the condition or to worsen it by altering their autoimmune system. Beauty therapists should not be encouraged to provide wax epilation over plaques (even though their clients find such exfoliation beneficial) without the client gaining permission from their medical advisor.

camouflage

application of fixing spray over the set skin camouflage may help to keep the camouflage in place and reduce any plaque shedding.

Camouflage can settle between the squames, making total removal difficult (it is suggested that you create the skin match on skin unaffected by psoriasis). A complementary colour is rarely needed. An even application is achieved when joints (such as elbows, knees, and knuckles) are flexed.

Some people may prefer to apply an emollient under camouflage because the plaques are usually very dry (the area can feel hot because the capillaries are closer to the surface).

rosacea

an inflammatory skin condition that is often associated with sun damage that primarily affects the face. In rare cases it can also affect the neck and chest. The exact cause is not known. People with rosacea are predisposed to blushing and flushing although there appears to be no direct evidence that rosacea is primarily a vascular disorder: it seems that the main abnormality is in the dermis that surrounds blood vessels rather than the vessel walls themselves. Sebum secretion is normal. This condition is often associated with sun damage.

clinical features

characterised by frequent blushing or persistent facial erythema. Intermittently telangiectasia, papules, pustules and swelling may also present. In its severe form, the nose becomes swollen and bulbous. It usually affects people aged between 30 and 60, but can also be seen from the mid-teens. It primarily affects skin groups 1 to 3. Rosacea affects men and women equally.

Stage I

persistent facial erythema, telangiectasia is more obvious and presents on the nose, cheeks, forehead and chin. Skin may feel hot and uncomfortable.

Stage II

papules and pustules are evident and can last for weeks. Facial pores are larger and more prominent. Flushing continues and thread veins appear. Skin is generally very irritated and extremely sensitive to skin care products, cosmetics and toiletries, and in some cases water.

Stage III

the facial contours may become coarse, thickened and irregular with inflamed oedematous skin and the nose may become purple coloured and enlarged (rhinophyma). There is permanent redness to the face.

dispelling social myths

Many people suffer profound psychological distress - life can be very stressful when you have a red face. Shakespeare's reference to 'grog blossom' gives rise to a red face and rhinophyma being associated with alcoholism: something which can still be incorrectly assumed to be the cause or contributing factor of rosacea.

camouflage

because the rosacea areas are highly sensitive and prone to blushing the practitioner should avoid working on the area until a skin match has been agreed. Some may prefer to use camouflage that has no oil in its formulation although crème camouflage is not known to affect rosacea adversely. Very finely milled powders may block facial pores (Stage II rosacea) and contribute to papules and pustules. A complementary colour may be required to mask severe erythema.

scars

form where the skin has been cut by accident or deliberately, as in the case of surgery, ceremonial markings, fashionable scarification, self-harming or the result of a dermatosis (such as acne) or an illness (such as chickenpox). Scars also result from burn injuries.

clinical features to all scars

scar tissue may be atrophic, hypertrophic or keloid, with the colour being erythematous, hypopigmented or hyperpigmented. The skin will usually be drier (although appearing to shine) with hypersensitivity, especially to sunlight.

Skin graft tissue will feel and appear different in colour to the surrounding skin: it may be puckered and have less elasticity.

scar revision

new techniques are constantly being devised; there are several procedures that may improve scar tissue cosmetically. These include intralesional injections, cryotherapy (to reduce keloid) and dermabrasion/resurfacing. All resurfacing techniques aim to change the dermal profile, which is the cause of contour defects. However, scars cannot be totally removed; they can be altered, reshaped and reduced but you always substitute one scar for another.

Scars may be revised (altering the position of reducing the scar) usually after it has matured. This is important when the scar has tightened and is over a joint and restricting movement. "Z-plasty", "W-plasty", "V-Y advancement" and "jumping man" are all descriptive names for altering the direction and position of a scar. By changing their direction they may also be less visible.

Skin resurfacing by laser and surgical dermabrasion are techniques which remove the epidermis over areas of uneven scarring. These procedures may have a limited role to play in the overall management of scars, especially the deeper "ice-pick" scarring associated with acne. Hospitalisation with full general anaesthetic is required. The area then re-epithelises and heals in about 10 days. Erythema can be very apparent for many months and a total sunblock must be used continually for at least one to two years.

Micro-dermabrasion (exaggerated exfoliation) is a superficial treatment available from beauty salons and cosmetic clinics. The treatment removes the top layers from the surface of the corneum, which may temporarily reduce fine wrinkles and improve the skin's texture but has little effect on scars, solar lentigines and telangiectasia. IPL and laser systems are also often used for skin rejuvenation as they can help to improve the skin texture by stimulating the formation of collagen within the dermis.

dispelling social myths

facial scars can give an impression of violence or a violent nature. Neither may be true. A small scar causes the same psychological problems as large areas of scarring. Often the person will consider their scarring a greater psychological problem than its cause; parental guilt is a particular issue when a child is involved. In some communities scarring may also have a social stigma.

camouflage

avoid skin toners; consider applying a fine layer of sunblock just before the camouflage (this may also help the camouflage adhere to the scar tissue) and allow the camouflage to slip over the scarring without dragging the skin. Applying a porcelain colour camouflage before the skin match can help minimise shine and act as a complementary to erythema and hyperpigmentation. Excessive powdering may result in the area looking caked.

The person must seek medical opinion when there is any suspicious lesion in the margins of their scar and skin camouflage should be discontinued until medical diagnosis.

striae distensae (stretch marks)

is the result of changes in the connective tissue of the skin, often but wrongly blamed on pregnancy (striae gravidarum), that occur at sites of skin stretching. It is thought that the adrenal gland hormones (common in Cushing's Syndrome) cause striae. They can also be a side effect of topical steroids.

clinical features

these are linear marks that initially appear pink-red-purple but can later become silvery white. They are common in adolescent boys (on the thighs and buttocks), in pregnancy (on the breasts, buttocks, abdomen and thighs), and can also appear elsewhere after relatively rapid weight gain/loss.

dispelling social myths

it is untrue that only those formerly obese and pregnant women get stretch marks.

camouflage

it is easier and quicker for the person to cover the whole area, rather than laboriously camouflaging each stria. Erythema and silver-shine can be minimised (see scar camouflage above).

tattoos

occur when any pigmented material is introduced and trapped within the dermis, such as:

intentional

by Radiographers to identify treatment area and by medical tattoo practitioners to replace lips, brows, areola, etc.

accidental

as a direct result from a graze, road traffic accident, an explosion or scoring the skin with a pen/pencil/biro.

deliberate

skin decoration by self or professionally applied inks and dyes to the dermis.

clinical features

decorative tattoos may be single or multi-coloured, from simple to multi-complex designs. An allergic reaction can occur to the dye used and infection may occur because of unhygienic equipment (especially with self-applied tattoos). Mercury-based dyes (now rare) often give a hypertrophic reaction scar. Radiographers usually use black but can sometimes create a mark that resembles a mole or freckle.

dispelling social myths

the recent fashion trend has dispelled the previous social-character associations; however they are still considered by some to be a statement made by anti-social individuals.

camouflage

it is impractical to reproduce the design by using individual complementary colours. You will need to identify the predominant colour for complementary purposes. One complementary colour can then be used over the whole area, powdered and then sealed with fixing spray before applying the skin match. You may need two applications of skin match over the complementary.

Crème camouflage is the preferred format to use.

After a few hours tattoos can have the unfortunate habit of ghosting back through the camouflage. Advise the person accordingly and suggest that they might need to apply additional skin match camouflage more frequently.

telangiectases (thread veins and spider naevi)

are caused by the dilation of small, thin blood capillaries – single or multiple – usually on the face (upper cheeks, nose and orbital area) but may appear on the legs. The cause is generally unknown but is thought to have a genetic factor. It is more common in adults. Telangiectases sometimes appear alongside other dermatoses, such as scleroderma and rosacea, and can be one of the side effects of multiple steroid injections when treating keloid scarring.

clinical features
telangiectasia

present as multiple wavy red lines on the affected area.

spider naevus

has a central spot or body with smaller lines radiating from it resembling the legs of a spider. Spider angioma may appear larger than spider naevus to the face. Spider naevi can be a sign of underlying disease.

dispelling social myths

a ruddy face is often associated with those who work in the open air. However, it may be that the lack of sunscreens to combat extreme climate conditions and wind plays a major role in the development of symmetrical telangiectases. There is no general connection between lack of skin care and the appearance of telangiectases/spider naevi.

camouflage

it is easier and quicker for the person to cover the whole area, rather than laboriously camouflage each thread vein or spider 'leg'.

vitiligo and leucoderma

both have an absence of melanocytes within the epidermis. The cause of vitiligo is not known, but there have been significant advances in our understanding of the condition in recent years. There is undoubtedly a genetic aspect as vitiligo often runs in families; a study of twins showed that both identical twins are more likely to develop the condition than both non-identical twins are. Vitiligo is associated with disorders that are considered to be autoimmune, which implies that vitiligo may also be autoimmune in origin. Leucoderma is a generic term that can be caused by any trauma to the melanocytes.

clinical features
leucoderma

is asymmetrical and usually remains unchanged in shape, size and location.

vitiligo

often in a strikingly symmetrical pattern on both sides of the face and body. The lesions are usually well defined and can be any shape or size. It is common for the patches to change shape, size and location. It can affect people of all skin groups, of either gender and at any age. Some people develop universal vitiligo in which all natural pigment is lost. Around 10–20% of people experience a spontaneous return of their normal pigment to an area of vitiligo skin.

vitiligo alopecia

with this condition white patches can also appear in the hair, including eyebrows, eyelashes and body hair. This may also be called piebaldism.

special considerations

skin without melanin is extremely susceptible to burning in the sun and it is known that trauma to the skin, such as that caused by sunburn, can encourage the vitiligo to spread. Sunscreens should always be applied before outdoors, as well as reapplied throughout the day (sunscreen can be applied over crème skin camouflage).

dispelling social myths

vitiligo and leucoderma are not contagious. Loss of pigmentation can have social and psychological implications. Children often experience teasing and name-calling. Adults can also feel stigmatised. Since vitiligo has been known about for at least 5,000 years it is not surprising that many myths have developed about the condition. In some cultures vitiligo is associated with leprosy and although the two conditions are completely different the stigma remains. To have vitiligo in the family, even if it is only in a distant cousin, may be enough to prevent a marriage taking place.

Some people believe that eating two white foods together, for example milk and fish, will cause vitiligo or make it worse - there is no evidence to support this myth.

People are extremely conscious of lesions on their hands and face, and are always looking for satisfactory ways to disguise them. They do not want the added embarrassment of cosmetics coming off their hands onto the objects they touch. Depigmentation to the lips and to genitalia gives particular psychological-social problems to people as they can be incorrectly assumed to have a sexually transmitted infection. The use of tinted sunscreens or faux tans may be of help to those who do not wish to use skin camouflage.

camouflage

is less successful on the hands because of frequent contact with water and detergents. One solution is to encourage them to apply faux suntan products under camouflage, which will help to minimise stark areas of depigmented skin and also provide some visual colouration if the camouflage crème become patchy or dislodged. The faux tan needs to be applied some time before camouflage application (see individual manufacturers' guidelines for timeframe for colour to develop). While the correct depth of colour may not be achieved by this method, a tanned skin rather than depigmented skin can be psychologically more acceptable.

Products Available To Camouflage Hands (PATCH) enquiry. The purpose of this joint venture undertaken with the Vitiligo Society was to find out what products lasted longer than traditional skin camouflage when applied to backs of hands and fingers. We tried to make it as 'scientific' as possible, so that the results would be reliable. Products tested were decanted into plain containers, so that participants did not know what brand they were testing; and the person collating the results did not know this either. As might be expected, participants in the enquiry often had quite different experiences with the products, different views and different priorities for deciding whether they liked them or wanted to use them again.

However, it is possible to make some generalisations. The venture has been a resounding success - all the products lasted longer than traditional camouflage, in many cases for 2 days or more. Although not a comparative survey, the fake tans were particularly strong on this criterion. Analyses of individual products have been sent to the manufacturers. It is hoped that at least some of them will be persuaded by the findings to extend their colour range to include skin staining products to mimic natural colours for skin groups 1 to 6. The survey also highlighted specialist theatrical cosmetics were long lasting and rub proof – however, there is concern that because these are activated and removed by alcohol solutions they should not be frequently applied elsewhere, especially to the face.

xanthelasma

is a common form of xanthoma.

clinical features

the condition presents as yellow lesions over the eyelids or under the eye.

camouflage

if the yellowing is very pronounced, the skin match camouflage can be set with a hint of pink powder to combat sallowness.

medical tattooing :
an alternative to daily camouflage applications

by Dawn Cragg MBE

the results should be very convincing;
medical tattooing can be a long-term alternative to
daily skin camouflage or the "finishing touch" to surgery

medical tattooing – an alternative to daily camouflage applications

This chapter is designed to give you background information to advise those who could benefit from a more permanent method of skin camouflage. This form of tattooing (which is sometimes referred to as micropigmentation) can be used to implant colour into the dermis for a specific medical purpose, such as,

- create lips, adjust symmetry and colour to lips
- augment and create realistic eyebrows
- create the nipple-areola complex (NAC) following breast reconstruction
- replace natural skin colour to small areas of leucoderma
- create the impression of natural beard shadow to small areas of leucoderma

However, the term micropigmentation is perhaps more associated with cosmetic tattooing to achieve semi-permanent make-up, such as lip line and lip colour enhancement, eyebrow shaping and eye lining, which may create a false impression (with limits to its uses) and deter people from seeking advice. Whether accidental (when someone unintentionally marks their skin, for example with a pencil) or deliberately applied, any colour that is introduced into the dermis and remains there is effectively a tattoo. The word tattoo can cause a psychological barrier for people who associate that only with artistic decoration to the skin. Consequently some practitioners call themselves derma-graphic artists or intra-dermal repigmentation consultants.

is medical tattooing permanent?

medical tattoos to the face, neck and hands will fade because the skin is exposed to sunlight. How quickly this might happen is very individual; some would need to boost the colour every few months or so; others annually. For example, to maintain skin matching camouflage on a hypopigmented scar (for skin groups 1-3) they could require follow-up sessions annually. Pigments that are protected by clothing will last longer but can fade over time. Unfortunately, if an inexperienced technician penetrates the epidermis, then that pigment will desquamate very quickly - within a few weeks.

Black and very highly coloured medical tattoo pigments and inks used for decorative tattoos appear not to blanch, although with time they do because of exposure to sunlight and the colour migrating through the skin. When medical tattooing is used to create skin camouflage, less vivid, natural colours are used. Unfortunately, the more pastel then the quicker the colour can alter or fade.

Realistic results require the practitioner to have a good understanding of the products used and how to mix the pigments to achieve an acceptable colour. The technician will also need to be aware that the depth of implantation will alter the final result of all pigments.

Pigments used for cosmetic and medical tattooing should be implanted approximately 0.5 to 2mm into the dermis. Pigment implanted deeper into the dermis has greater longevity, but may be prone to unfavourable colour changes. However, people should be made aware that it is not desirable to have permanency because their skin and hair will fade over time and the medical tattoo will need to mirror those changes. An annual follow up procedure is usually required to maintain the colour.

There are many different types of pigment available for implantation. However, all pigments used for medical and cosmetic tattooing must be sourced from suppliers that manufacture under strict guidelines, complying with the EU Resolution Res AP(2008)1. These must not contain substances which endanger the health or safety of persons or the environment. They must be gamma sterilised, sold in tamper proof bottles (or unit dose phials) together with EU labelling requirements, as mentioned in page 21. Accompanying Material Safety Data Sheet(s) must be readily available for reference to check exactly what is in each and every bottle of colour. Other countries may have different regulations concerning components used. The black dye paraphenylenedeamine (PPD) is a known sensitizer, and not used in cosmetic and medical tattooing pigments.

The product has a larger molecular structure (micron count) than inks used for decorative tattoos and are, therefore, the preferred products for safe and realistic cosmetic and medical tattooing. The powder colour(s) are combined in dispersion – a solution such as propylene glycol, distilled water and isopropyl alcohol. It is essential to colour test the pigment on the surface of the person's skin before proceeding with the tattooing.

inorganic pigments
are composed of insoluble metallic compounds most commonly iron oxides. They are not made from natural sources, and have good stability. Colours are from the earthy dusky palettes, such as ochre (mustard colours) and reds (brick colours), which will fade with time

organic pigments
are from the bright vibrant colour palettes (bright reds, oranges and yellows) and do not dissolve as well as iron oxides when missed with hydration products. There have been some listed cases of allergic reaction to organic pigments.

inks
are fully soluble colours traditionally used by decorative tattoo artists. Colours are implanted deeper into the reticular dermis and are permanent; however, colours will fade with time and UV exposure.

contraindications
tattooing is contraindicated in the following circumstances,
- should they have unrealistic expectations of the outcome
- for people with dysmorphophobia
- on any areas of infection
- an allergic reaction to the pigments and inks used
- over any hyperpigmentation (any marks that are darker to the surrounding skin colour)
- on erythema (any lesion which is more red than the surrounding skin colour)
- on keloid scars
- on hypertrophic and erythematous scarring
- over freckles and age spots
- on moles or any suspicious looking lesions
- on acne "ice-pick" scars
- on varicose veins, thread-veins and spider naevi
- over port wine stains and strawberry birthmarks
- on under eye circles of discoloured skin
- to cover a tribal, decorative or cosmetic tattoos
- over very delicate skin grafts
- over stretch marks covering a large area (because it is impossible to make a significant improvement)
- if the person is pregnant
- on someone who has acquired a tan (faux or sun)

You must also ensure that there are no further reconstructive procedures planned, which could distort or alter the placement of the medical tattoo. The medical tattoo will need to be protected should they consider IPL and LASER procedures. GB law prohibits the application of decorative tattoos on minors, but there is no age restriction when the procedure is deemed for a medical reason and requested by the child's medical advisor. The technician must be insured for such work and the procedure undertaken with the child's adult representative present.

Medical tattooing cannot be used to remove colour from an existing tattoo or from hyperpigmented lesions.

It is prudent that people gain consent for medical tattooing to proceed from their medical advisor. However, it might not be necessary to obtain such permission for aesthetic (cosmetic) lip and eye enhancement tattooing.

code of practice

a patch test to determine an allergic reaction is compulsory. The technician's failure to comply with this will result in the cancellation of insurance. Iron oxide pigments should be tested for 24 hours. Organic pigments should be tested for 30 days as these are the ones most likely to cause a reaction. Should the patch test be negative but an allergic reaction occur later, then no treatment can be given until medical opinion is sought. There are known cases of secondary reactions, sometimes years later; therefore a patch test is also required prior to any annual "top-up." The technician must always be aware and not assume no reaction will take place.

Although the position of the technician to the patient is a personal choice, the person should always be in a semi-upright position during facial tattooing. If the person is lying flat on the couch, the facial muscles can distort and when seated upright again the tattooed area could look uneven or wrong. The same principle applies for NAC, however, people can can be repositioned once the outline has been drawn.

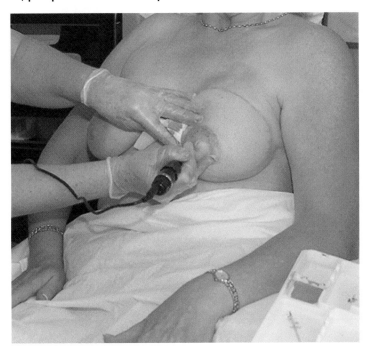

02 *patient in a semi-upright position*
Dawn Cragg, BASC Member 2151

It is essential that the technician discusses in full and the person totally approves of the depth of colour, size and shape of the suggested treatment. The technician must adopt an empathetic role, which empowers people with the decision making. Such an interaction will also be therapeutic and should form a strong professional bond between them and the technician. No work should commence until the person signs agreement on the consent form.

After a thorough consultation the technician will need to take and record good quality "before" photographs of the person. Photographs should also be taken and recorded on completion of each treatment.

All equipment used in GB must conform to EU standards with disposable cartridges. A machine with Class 2a certification is preferable as this can be used in an operating theatre - should there be a need for a surgeon (or qualified technician) to use medical tattooing when the person is under general anaesthetic.

conditions where medical tattooing is successful

the more skin discolouration there is in an area the easier it is to disguise and the more natural the end result can be for procedures such as,

camouflaging hypopigmented scars and skin grafts

creating a natural skin colour is more successful on flat scars. The success of medical tattooing to camouflage skin grafts depends on the condition of the skin and the strength of the graft – it may be that the area is too delicate. It is not advisable to work on any graft or scar until it has matured, which would be at least one year old. If a scar remains erythematous, medical opinion should be sought to see if silicone dressings, LASER treatment or another procedure could improve the colour prior to starting any medical tattoo procedure.

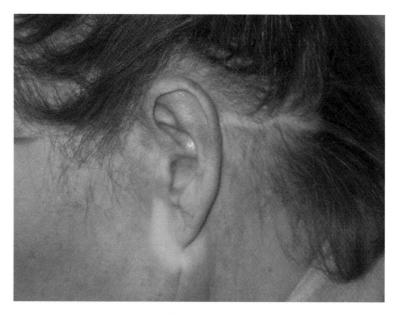

scarring around ear

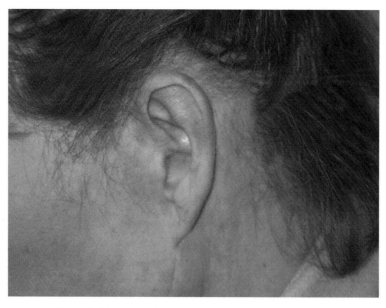

tattooed skin matching colour to camouflage the scar
© Tarryn Vice, Finishing Touches

150

repigmentation to vitiligo and leucoderma lesions

people must be made fully aware of problems that can occur when adding colour to hypopigmented lesions. They must also be advised that the added colour will fade and that they should be prepared to return for regular annual colour boosting. Unfortunately the colour added may unwittingly create discolouration or a less than satisfactory result.

Although vitiligo may be in remission, people can wake up to find white halos around the site of repigmentation. Research is ongoing as to why medical tattooing can trigger the return of vitiligo.

creating and repigmenting the nipple and areola

medical tattooing eliminates the need for someone to use a prosthetic nipple. It is also very successful in creating a nipple and areola following reconstruction surgery and to enhance natural colour where pigment is missing. Trompe l'oeil (3D effects) can be used to create the illusion of protrusion of a raised nipple by adding shadows and highlights.

All surgery must be complete and the reconstruction breast allowed to settle into a natural shape, which is a minimum of 6 months post procedure. Any further surgery in the breast area could result in distortion of the areola and nipple.

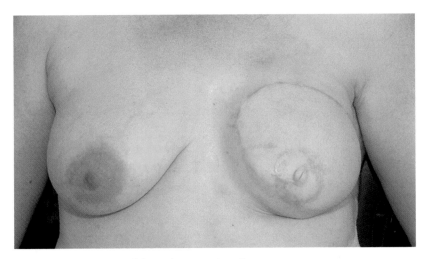

02 post reconstructive surgery

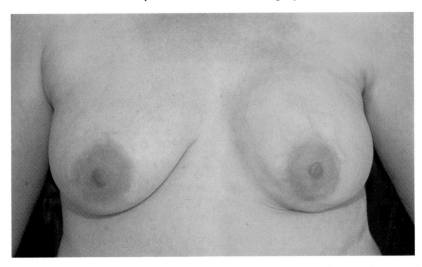

02 tattooed natural colours to the nipple and areola and a false vein to match
that on the other breast; skin matching camouflage to the scarring
Dawn Cragg, BASC Member 2151

creating and reshaping lips

medical tattooing to outline and colour the lips is particularly recommended for those who,

- have lost partial or full lip definition following reconstructive surgery
- have naturally uneven shape to their lip
- have lost the colour to their lips
- have thin lips

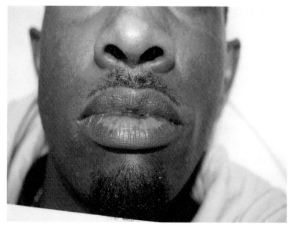

lower lip hypopigmentation
© Gail Proudman, Finishing Touches

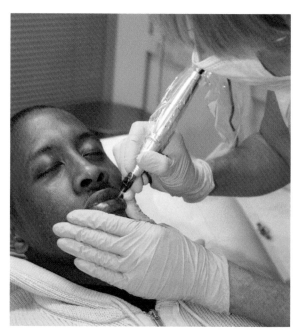

the tattoo treatment in progress
© Gail Proudman, Finishing Touches

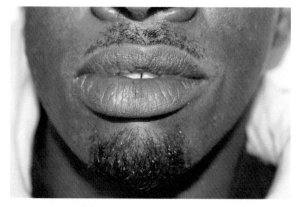

natural lip colour tattooed to lower lip
© Gail Proudman, Finishing Touches

creating hair simulation

sparse growth or total loss of hair is particularly stressful when it affects facial hair. Medical tattooing can be used to,

create eyebrows in a hair-by-hair technique on people
- undergoing chemotherapy
- who have permanent alopecia
- post reconstruction surgery

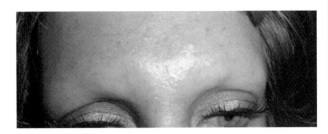

alopecia to brow
© Dawn Cragg, BASC Member 2151

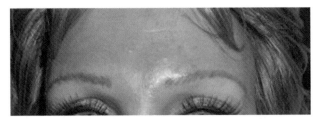

unless the patient requests differently,
the tattoo must represent brow hairs
© Dawn Cragg, BASC Member 2151

The hair-by-hair technique is preferable to add bulk and colour for people who have over-tweezed their eyebrows

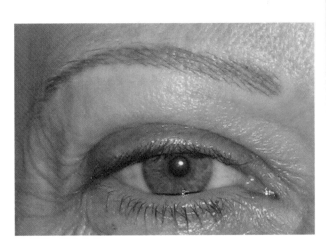

adding bulk to over tweezed brow
© Kelly Forshaw, Finishing Touches

Colour can be introduced to give definition to eyes for those who have no eyelashes and add faux stipple to beard shadow when scarring interferes with natural growth

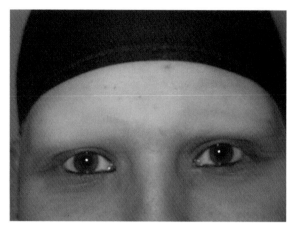

with tattooed eyeliner
© Kelly Forshaw, Finishing Touches

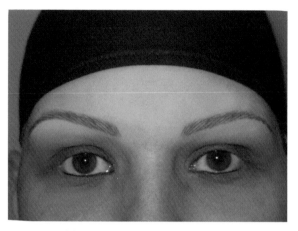

with tattooed brows and eyeliner
© Kelly Forshaw, Finishing Touches

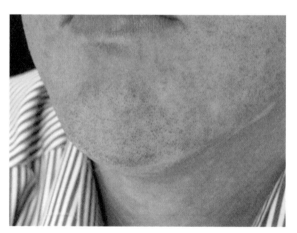

alopecia (scarring) to beard growth
© Dawn Cragg, BASC Member 2151

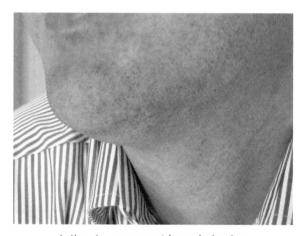

tattoo to represent beard shadow
© Dawn Cragg, BASC Member 2151

Medical tattooing to stipple colour can be successful when applied to very small scars but it is not recommended for people who have natural balding, skin grafts, alopecia and dermatoses that present widespread scalp hair loss.

scar relaxation (also known as dermarolling)

this involves using a dry needle technique called Micro-Needling to break down the bands of connective tissue that otherwise can produce tightening and deformity of the skin. The result is a smoother and flatter scar. Usually this technique is applied at a separate appointment, however, for small scars (such as in the eyebrow or on the lip line) the scar will often relax and flatten as the medical tattooing takes place.

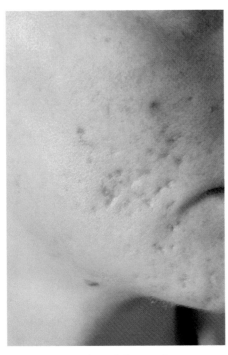

acne ice-pick scarring
© Helen Porter, Finishing Touches

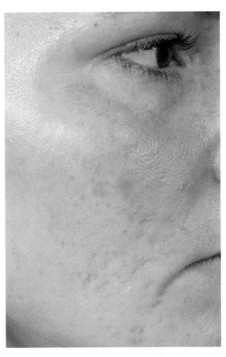

post scar relaxation (dry-needling) treatment
© Helen Porter, Finishing Touches

Scar relaxation is not recommended for everyone and people must be advised to seek opinion and permission from their medical practitioner before agreeing to this method of treatment.

what can go wrong?

it is important to choose a specialist technician who is well trained and has accumulated a wealth of experience. The following mistakes could occur when the technician is inexperienced,

- poor foundation knowledge of colour selection
- inappropriate choice of colour used
- pigment migration due to incorrect needle insertion or the needle being inserted too deeply
- maceration of skin tissue by overworking the area
- unsymmetrical lip borders
- uneven eye liner
- incorrect placement of eyebrows (too high or too low)
- unflattering shape of eyebrows (too long, too short)

referring people for a medical tattoo consultation

unfortunately at the time of going to print the medical tattooing and micropigmentation profession is unregulated. It is therefore vital you obtain background knowledge of the technician and ask the following questions,

- is a licence needed in the area in which the person is working?
- If a licence is required, have they got one?
- how long have they been in practice?
- how long have they practised medical tattooing?
- did the technician qualify with an accredited specialist training provider?
- who are the insurers?

You are entitled to request and be shown a copy of their insurance policy and local authority licence. And, most importantly, ask for medical references and testimonials from their previous work!

training opportunities

anyone who advertises as a training school must have an exemplary reputation in this specialism and that the graduate's qualification will be recognised by NHS professionals, hospitals, local authorities and insurance companies. The tutor must be an expert and possess evidence of recent continuing professional development. The trainee needs to confirm that they will be taught using equipment and products that comply with EU regulations and that all knowledge and technology will be up-to-date. A typical training programme requires the student to be competent in aesthetic (cosmetic) techniques before training in the skills necessary to provide a medical tattoo service. Medical professionals can elect to learn medical tattooing techniques on the body as a stand alone diploma, but if they wish to treat other areas then they should consider learning aesthetic tattooing techniques prior to learning facial medical tattooing procedures.

The trainee should take the following precautionary steps before committing to a training programme:

- check the tutor is insured to teach the procedures you wish to learn
- check that you will be able to get insurance for yourself once you have completed your training
- check that the trainer has a licence to practice
- ask to view the tutor's portfolio and verify their references
- ask to visit the place of training before you sign any contract
- ask to see the tutor's certificates and diplomas, especially those for continuing professional development.

It is vital that the course is a mixture of theory and hands-on practice on a wealth of models.

9

postiche, prostheses and false nails

Health is a state of complete physical, mental and social well-being
And not merely the absence of disease or infirmity.

World Health Organisation
Mental Health Fact Sheet No. 220 : Sept 2010

postiche, prostheses and false nails

This section is designed to give you background information on items that people might be wearing, or may consider using to enhance their appearance or replace something which is temporarily or permanently lost. Do not make a direct suggestion to them that they should wear postiche, prosthesis or false nails as many prefer not to. However you should be aware of local specialists who can help, because people may ask your advice on who can provide these services as well as cleaning and replacing items.

facial postiche
the major function of eyelashes and eyebrows is to protect the eye and brow bone. It is their absence that causes concern to people because their face loses its framework around the eye area and, to a greater extent, expression and visual facial emotion are lost.

lashes
eyelashes have an approximate four-month growth cycle, reaching an average maximum length of 1.25cm (½"). At the time of going to print, skin grafts (hair transplants) to create eyelashes have yet to be perfected. In the absence of natural eyelashes, it may be better to use a decorative cosmetic (or medical tattooing) to outline the eye and give the impression that a lash line exists. Where lash growth is sparse, postiche (false) lashes can be applied.

postiche eye lashes
are available as single (individual lashes) or in continuous strips that are applied with special adhesive and removed by solvents designed for that purpose (no other glue or solvents should be used). Always follow the manufacturer's instructions and not allow adhesive or solvent to come into contact with eyes. Contraindications include inflamed or swollen lids, of if the person has an eye disorder such as conjunctivitis or blepharitis. People may be allergic to the adhesive and solvent.

Individual lashes are not reusable after application and removal whereas strip lashes can be used several times before they become spent. People soon learn how to apply their own strip lashes but individual lashes may need to be applied by a qualified therapist.

individual lashes
are glued to the base of an existing eyelash to make that individual lash hair appear more full. They are also used to infil a space in the lash line by attaching single lashes to natural ones either side of the gap. Their main advantage is that they do not need to be removed daily. They tend to last several days (adhesion continuing) and could remain in place as long as the lash is attached to its follicle. This form of postiche can be considered more natural looking as the lashes adhere to existing lashes and not the eyelid skin.

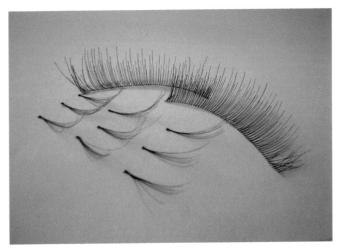

03 examples of strip and individual lashes

strip lashes
are single lashes glued to a base strip, which is adhered to the edge of the eyelid and designed to sit on top of the existing lashes. Obvious care must be taken when placing strip lashes so that there is no 'tramline' effect. This form of postiche needs to be removed daily. Although the lashes can be reapplied directly, people may have to clean them carefully first. Where people have a gap in the lash line which does not require full strips, you can trim off the required length.

eyebrows

brow hair has a growth cycle of up to four months and grows to an average length of 1.25cm (½"). At the time of going to print, hair transplant (sometimes using the person's pubic, instead of scalp hair) is proving successful.

postiche brows

pre-made theatrical brow postiche, where human or synthetic hair is vented (knotted) onto a fine net base, is available from specialist retailers. Other forms of facial postiche (beards, moustaches and sideburns) are made in the same way. The hair-free margin of the net base is glued to the skin. While these items are excellent for theatrical purposes, they are not considered practical normal wear as the net would be visible.

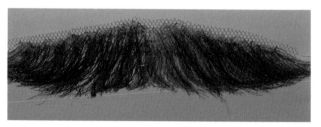

theatrical moustache illustrating the net margin

Similarly, crepe hair is no longer considered a convincing solution to facial hair loss.

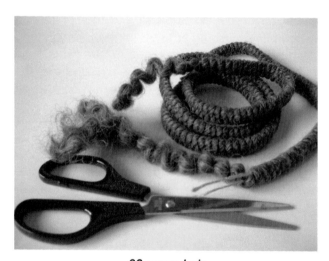

03 crepe hair

Pencilling in missing brow hairs is a simple remedy, as is creating a whole pencilled brow (see page 90 for brow shapes and application techniques). Medical tattoo brow hairs may be considered for people not suitable for grafts.

demi and full scalp postiche

scalp hair can reach a length of 100cm or more during its seven year growth cycle. On average the hair grows 1.25cm (½") a month but that process will slow with age, illness and some medications. Growth cycle varies considerably for different individuals. An average head will naturally shed approximately 100 hairs each day from the 100,000 to 150,000 present on the scalp.

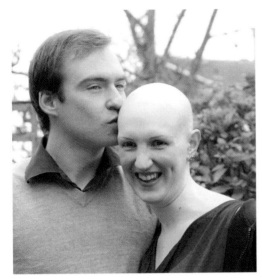 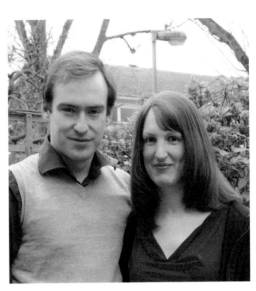

Vicky (founder of Alopecia UK) and friend
© Alopecia UK

While the function of head hair is to protect the scalp from UV irradiation and help prevent heat loss, there is a great psychological need for us to have head hair. We are all aware of how rotten we feel when we have a 'bad hair day' and immediately feel uplifted after our hair is washed, cut or coloured and finished in a fashionable style. To lose part, or all, of one's hair (whatever the cause) can have a devastating effect on people's self-esteem.

The term demi postiche is used to describe any hairpiece that does not cover the whole head, such as hair extensions and a male toupee; full scalp postiche means a full wig.

creating scalp postiche
there are two methods of creating demi and full scalp postiche.

The first is by weaving hair into weft lengths, which are then sewn onto special ribbon (galloon) to create the required piece. Machines have replaced this once labour intensive method, with synthetic hair usually used instead of human. This makes the cost of manufacture and retail very low. Synthetic hair has the advantage that the piece can easily be rinsed through and, being pre-set, will not require much after-care attention. The negative side to synthetic hair is that the piece can be hot to wear and the colour and texture of the hair may not appear very natural. Wefted postiche is usually sold as a standard sized piece, requiring the wearer to adjust the tension springs to reduce the size to fit snugly.

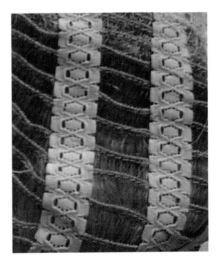

03 wefted postiche, with weft attached to the galloon ribbon

Postiche made from micro-fibre synthetic hair is more expensive but being heat resistant allows the person to use a hairdryer and heated curling appliances. Micro-fibre postiche looks like natural hair and is comfortable to wear; it can be constructed by either wefting or venting.

Vented human hair postiche can require more care and attention, will be cooler to wear and can be exceptionally convincing. Most human hair postiche require specialist dry cleaning but some can be 'washed and dried' at home or cleaned by a local hairdresser. The price paid for the postiche will depend on the cost, quantity and the length of the hair used and the time taken by the posticheur to knot the hair into the net base by hand. This form of postiche is usually tailor-made to fit the wearer and measurements are taken at the time of ordering.

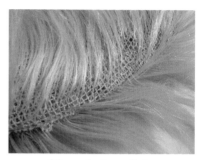

03 vented postiche

Also available for people with total scalp hair loss (alopecia totalis or universalis alike) are vented postiche to a silicone foundation (cap) tailor-made to fit the individual's head. The cap creates a vacuum seal and secure fitment without the use of adhesive (toupee tape or glue) or mechanical attachment (clips or tension bands). However, this form of postiche is not suitable for people with remaining scalp hair because the hair could interfere with the vacuum seal and therefore compromise the attachment of the postiche to the head.

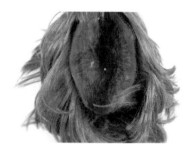

inside view of a custom made vented silicone postiche © Karena Moore-Millar

handling postiche

there is no need for people to remove their postiche during a camouflage consultation. However, camouflage will adhere to the hair and care must be taken not to soil the postiche. Do not attempt to push the postiche back from the forehead as this may result in the securing mechanism tearing the weft or vent net. If someone wishes to remove their postiche, allow them to handle the piece by holding it at the tension springs (not the hair itself) and place it on a wig tree until the end of the session.

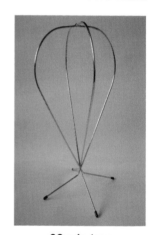

03 wig tree

Irrespective of which form the person chooses, all new postiche may need trimming to suit the individual's hairstyle. People should always be advised to take their postiche to a qualified hairdresser who is used to working with postiche. People can become concerned that fit and tension springs do not always prevent accidental movement during wear. The solution is to wear a wig-cap and secure the postiche to that with hairgrips. For additional security, double-sided toupee tape can be used to secure the wig-cap to the scalp (the weft and venting could tear if the tape was placed directly on the postiche).

Hair extensions which are secured direct to existing hair are an alternative to wearing postiche. It is also possible to secure (by sewing, gluing or weaving onto the surrounding hair) vented demi postiche. These methods require people to attend their specialist hairdresser at frequent intervals to maintain the postiche. Human and synthetic hair attached to a fine band are also available, which allows people to manage temporary hair extensions.

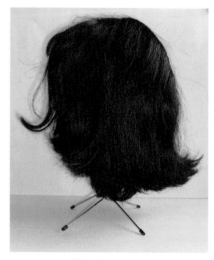

03 wig on tree

prosthetics

a prosthesis is any synthetic structure which in some way reproduces and replaces the natural biological human form. The role of the maxillofacial department is to provide a large range of dental prosthetics, including crowns, bridges and dentures. However some hospital Prosthesists will also create facial and body prostheses which may include many types of

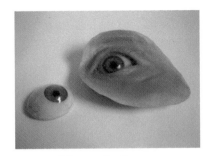

*03 prosthetic eye
and ocular prosthesis
including upper cheek*

- artificial limbs – including hands and fingers
- facial and body prostheses – including eyes, ears, noses, hands, fingers, nipples

There has been some success (especially when worn under hosiery) in using a made to measure prosthetic plug to infil severe atrophy. Suitability remains individual and upon the advice of the doctor. At the time of going to print there has been some success with prosthetic eyebrows and it is hoped that further advances will be made.

Prosthetics used to be made from silicone rubber; this was because its flexibility allowed it to bend to some extent with the natural movements of soft tissue and because of its lifelike appearance. Its disadvantages are that it attracts dirt easily, especially from its medical adhesive; it attracts nicotine from cigarette smoke and turns yellow; if exposed to strong sunlight it will bleach; and in time it will ultimately harden and lose flexibility. Because of these disadvantages, care, maintenance and periodical reconstruction were necessary and of great importance. New technologies include the use of CT scanners and digital recording of someone's skeletal deformity. From this information a very accurate skeletal model can be made using a computer/robot controlled LASER shone into a bath of light cured resin; layer by layer this builds up any desired shape or component.

Retention is achieved by using modern medical adhesives which are more user and prosthesis friendly. Prosthetic nipples can be secured to skin with petroleum jelly or by directly inserting between bra and breast.

During the 1980s it was discovered that a highly refined grade of titanium could be made to bond with living bone. This development allows medical grade titanium implants to be placed into facial bone; intern clips are then attached to the implants and the prosthesis attaches to the clips.

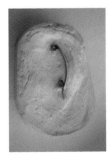

*03 titanium bar which is
implanted into the skull*

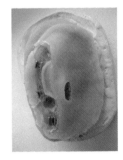

*03 intern clips attached
to reverse of prosthesis*

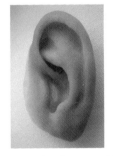

*03 prosthetic ear, with
hole to facilitate hearing,
ready to clip into place*

camouflage and prostheses

camouflage products do not usually adhere to prosthetics, so the skills of maxillofacial technicians also include colouring the item to match the person's skin. The margin between prosthesis and natural skin can be blended together (if required) by a light application of camouflage, using a stipple sponge, of the chosen skin match.

It is not usually necessary for the person to remove their prosthesis during a skin match consultation. However, always expect the unexpected, never show shock or surprise, and handle prostheses with due respect and care.

false nails and nail extensions

on average, fingernails grow at a rate of ⅛" per month; toenail growth is slower. Hands, like faces, are nearly always on show, and the way a person is treated can be affected by the appearance of their hands.

If there is a problem with the hand itself – such as psoriasis, scarring, vitiligo – paying attention to clean and manicured nails may be a way of drawing the eye away from the dermatosis or scar.

Damaged nails can have an adverse affect on others. For instance, a condition may be thought of as contagious or dirty and, as hands are used for touch, others may in ignorance shy away. There are many reasons why nails are damaged. The most likely reasons are

- Onychomycosis: fungal infection of the nail plate. There are several types; the most serious form destroys the layers of the nail plate.
- Onychoptosis: the loss of one or more nails; usually the result of disease or injury.
- Onychoxis: an overgrowth or thickening of the nail plate. Can be hereditary or a sign of stress or infection.
- Paronychia: an acute infection. This usually attacks people who have their hands constantly in water. It is a yeast infection which causes redness, swelling, pain and often oozing pus. It usually attacks only one or two nails.
- Tinea ungium (ringworm): this is a contagious disease caused by a vegetable parasite. The ringworm invades the free edge and spreads towards the matrix. Usually requires oral medication over several months to treat it.

All the above conditions should be referred to a doctor.

- Eczema: only affects the nail in extreme cases - if any broken skin surrounds the nail plate, referral to a GP is advisable.
- Leukonychia: these are white spots on the nail plate usually occurring in nails that are weak or delicate. The main cause is external injury which, in turn, causes a separation in the nail cells and allows air to permeate the cells. Can also be caused through a build-up of acid that collects under the cuticle.
- Onychophagi: severe nail biting. This habit is responsible for a large number of nail deformities and can be accompanied by bitten skin surrounding the nail, leaving it red, open and sore.
- Psoriasis: when nails have been affected they can appear pitted, thickened or discoloured.

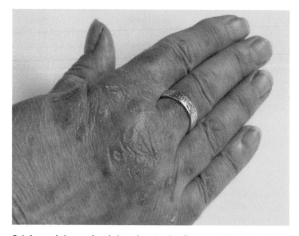

01 hand (psoriasis) prior to before nail extensions

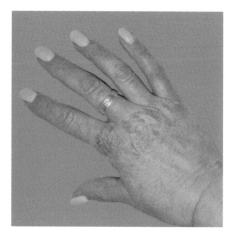

01 hand after nail extensions applied

With advancing technology, originally borrowed from the dental industry, help is now available in the shape of nail enhancements (false nails).

Nail conditions in the first group opposite are not suitable for false nails. Likewise, nails cannot be attached where there is no nail plate at all, especially so for toes. However, provided there is no infection, contagion or pain, nails can be disguised. The simplest method, of course, is to apply nail polish to the existing nail, although this may not be suitable for everyone. Buffing the nails to a high shine is an alternative.

Nail enhancements primarily come in two categories – sculpted and tips with overlay. The nail technician will normally diagnose which type is suitable for the condition of the nails and lifestyle of the wearer. Both males and females may wear nail enhancements. Frequent visits to the salon are required to infil the gap created between the natural nail growth and the false nail.

sculpted
sculpted means that a free edge is attached to the existing nail using a polymer resin liquid and powder. When dry this is then filed and shaped to look like a natural nail.

tips with overlay
most nail technicians use tips with overlay for speed and durability. A nylon or acrylic nail tip is glued on to the end of the existing nail, filed to a natural nail shape and buffed flush with the nail plate. An overlay is then placed over the tip and nail for strength and shape. Overlays commonly used are polymer resin liquid and powder, fibreglass resin and gels, which are mainly light cured.

care
before enhancements are attached, the technician will ensure that the nail plate is clean by wiping with an anti-fungal and antiseptic preparation. Nail enhancements should not damage the natural nail – only bad nail technicians can do that. A softening of the nail may be experienced when they are removed. False nails are soaked off with a special remover, pulling off will most certainly damage the nail plate.

People can purchase over-the-counter false nail kits, but the results do not last as long as nails applied professionally. They can also be the cause of fungal infections as they rarely contain adequate cleansing preparations or information. However, these are suitable for short-term use or in an emergency.

using decorative cosmetics (make-up) in conjunction with camouflage

the most important consideration is that the colour of the make-up does not reintroduce the colour of the dermatosis or scarring as this can psychologically remind people of what lies below and render their skin camouflage ineffective

using decorative cosmetics in conjunction with camouflage

One question you may be asked is "will make-up go over the camouflage?" People will be reassured to know that the simple answer is "yes!"

Make-up can also be used to great effect as a distraction - someone with attractively made-up eyes will draw attention away from a dermatosis or scar lower on the face; equally, someone with beautiful lips will divert focus from the eye area. However, there are a few cautions of which to be aware, both with the decorative colours and the products used. It may be that this advice is given during a later consultation after the initial camouflage application session, or it may play an important part during your first meeting.

You should not apply make-up to anyone unless you are qualified to do so. The following guidelines are designed to help you advise them about the best way to achieve their make-up application when used in conjunction with skin camouflage. It might be wise to keep a small range of coloured cosmetics (as suggested under each heading below) so that the person can understand and appreciate your recommendations.

Decorative cosmetics have identical contraindications to camouflage application and an allergic reaction to any product must be treated as previously discussed. People may not be aware that "use before" and "PAO" dates are applicable to their toiletries and cosmetics too. Hygienic, safe working practices and storage of items are the same as those for camouflage products and cosmetic applicators. You may also need to reaffirm the importance of preventing product contamination and deterioration.

The person needs to be made aware that their make-up should be applied with appropriate brushes, sponges and puffs – and not with fingers. This is especially important when applying decorative cosmetics over skin camouflage. The lightest touch is required otherwise the make-up could merge with, or disturb, the camouflage products underneath. Unless otherwise stated below, it is better to keep make-up brushes independent of camouflage brushes – although they may be an identical set.

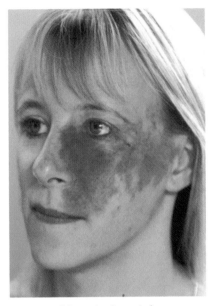

01 port wine stain

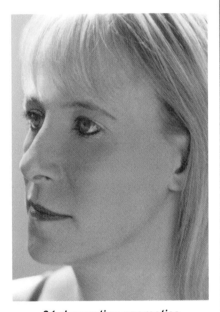

01 decorative cosmetics can be used in conjunction with skin camouflage

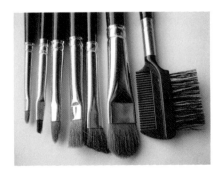

03 selection of make-up brushes and applicators

Decorative cosmetics cannot be successfully applied when the person is lying on a couch – they need to sit facing a mirror in good lighting. People (including you) should never use a magnifying mirror, as there is the temptation to apply too much. Brand loyalties are very individual, but once the product is on the face, that knowledge becomes unknown and irrelevant. The main criteria for any decorative cosmetic is,

- does the colour look good on me?
- do I like the texture and smell of the product?
- will it suit my budget?

There should be little, or no reason for people to stop using their favourite cosmetics but they may need to change the colours used and their application technique.

concealers

are mainly used to conceal shadows around the eyes, which become more apparent as we get older simply because the skin becomes thinner, and to areas of facial skin discoloration and erythema. Before using a concealer consider whether a skin match camouflage would give a better result. This is especially so if the person is using camouflage elsewhere – people can then use their camouflage without having to purchase another product. If the person wishes to also apply cosmetic foundation, they will need to check whether the manufacturer recommends that the concealer be applied before or after the foundation. Treat the area delicately, especially around the eye otherwise the delicate skin will not be able to hold the product.

product choice
concealers can be complementary or skin coloured and are sold usually in solid crème format, as a liquid or as tinted powders.

skin coloured concealer
unless you choose the correct skin match, you can unintentionally produce the opposite effect. If you apply a shade of concealer under the eye that is too light, the dark shadows will become a dull shade that is just as noticeable as it was before you applied anything.

complementary coloured concealer
it is better to try a skin coloured concealer first but if that does not camouflage the discolouration then people will need to use a complementary colour before applying foundation. Generally yellows are used as complimentary over red and blue undertones: pinks and mauves as complementary to brown shadows and sallow complexions. White and pale green concealers can create the same ghosting effects as with camouflage.

application technique
concealer is applied by either dotting onto the area or by following the line of discolouration; carefully blend with a fingertip, sponge or brush. The best method to ensure correct placement for under eye shadows is to point your chin towards your sternum and look up into a mirror.

cosmetic foundation

at the time of going to print, the British Association of Skin Camouflage has not received any reports that foundations, when used in conjunction with camouflage, change colour. However, there is the potential for the two products to mix together and create a different colour when the camouflage and foundation are not correctly applied.

You should advise people that they have the choice to carefully apply their foundation on top of the set crème camouflage, or apply crème or powder camouflage products over the foundation, or to apply foundation (any format) only to non-camouflaged skin.   Whichever method is chosen they will need to ensure that the products match in colour and is blended well at any margin between camouflage and foundation.

product choice
the quantity of pigment, water, oil and other ingredients in foundation formulations will vary from brand to brand – and differ from the slightest hint of colour to what can be as effective as camouflage. Someone with dry skin may benefit more from a crème foundation, whereas those with an oily skin should use a formulation that does not encourage their skin to shine quickly.

using camouflage as foundation
the easiest option is for people to blend their crème or powder camouflage over the whole of the face rather than applying an additional cosmetic. However, some people may feel that is too concealing for their normal look, in which case camouflage crème can be diluted by mixing a small amount of moisturiser with it before applying to non-camouflaged skin. The whole face then requires setting with powder.

foundation over camouflage
people may find it easier to use a liquid (mousse or cream-to-powder) foundation or a micro-mineral powder camouflage as these are less likely to disturb the set crème camouflage. The most common types of foundation do not usually require an application of powder as they "dry out" matt on the skin. The lightest possible touch is required, otherwise the camouflage crème could be dragged from its required place.

foundation under camouflage
those who prefer to apply their foundation before the camouflage product may choose either a liquid or crème formulation (micro-mineral powder is not recommended under a crème camouflage). Crème foundation will require setting with powder before their camouflage is applied.

application technique
this method gives an even application and allows careful blending and, most importantly, will not disturb any camouflage crème or foundation. Use a cosmetic sponge to "press and roll" the foundation onto the face, rather than use large sweeping movements.   A specialist application brush can be used when applying micro-mineral powder camouflage.

powder
before applying, check that the foundation requires it, as many do not.

product choice
for setting foundation/concealer it is better for people to use the same setting powder as used over their camouflage application, otherwise the finished look may be patchy and uneven.

application technique
this is an identical method as for setting camouflage and the powder puff can be the same one as used for setting their camouflage.

eyebrows

for those who have some eyebrow hair it is better to use a suitable coloured eye shadow or very soft brow pencil when working over skin camouflage, taking care not to drag the skin or disturb any camouflage underneath

product choice

however, for people who have eyebrow hairs lighter in colour than the others, you could suggest that they get their eyebrows tinted professionally, but if this is not available, use a mascara wand to colour match the affected hairs.

application technique

work from the temple (not the nose) end of the eyebrow, and carefully lift the hairs off the skin as you apply a fine layer of mascara. Wait a few seconds for it to dry, and then use a clean eyebrow comb to comb the hairs back into their natural line of growth. Going in the opposite direction to the natural growth ensures that no mascara ends up on the person's skin and the end result is extremely convincing. Depending on people's lifestyle, and potential to smudge the area, it may be better to use waterproof mascara.

If the person has fine brow hairs, mascara that is designed to give extra length and thicken may be the solution (using the application method described above)

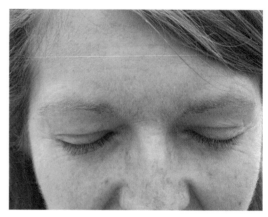

03 brows with thinning growth

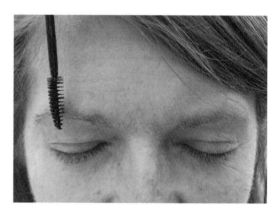

03 mascara wand lifting hairs

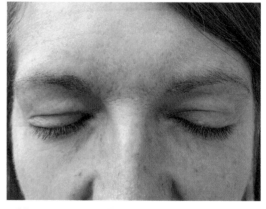

03 mascara applied to person's right brow

eye shadows

eyes also benefit from eye shadow colours being carefully mirrored under the lower lashes – it helps to make the eyes appear larger and prevents the camouflage/foundation colour and white of the eye merging.

product choice

crème formulated eye shadows require a powder application to set – but however many times powdering is used, the colours always seem to migrate to the socket crease. For that reason, and because they could merge with underlying camouflage, crème eye shadow is not the first product of choice in this context.

Soft and hard pencil eye shadows may drag the eyelid and could disturb any camouflage underneath.

Liquid (usually sold in pen format) and compressed powder format eye shadows work best over set camouflage.

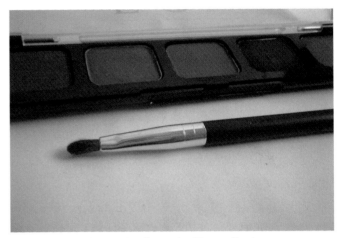

03 powder format with applicator

For someone with excessive tears or watering eyes, it might be useful to use skin staining or waterproof eye make-up. The person will need to practice using these: a little goes a long way and they need to be carefully blended with a dampened brush to give good results. This variety of eye make-up (including shadow, liner and mascara) will need to be removed with a cleanser that will easily remove the product without irritating the skin or eye.

application technique

eye shadow applicators and brushes come in an assortment of shapes and sizes. A soft bristle brush gives the best results. Whether it is contoured, square or round shaped is personal choice. People will need to apply their eye shadow using gentle brush stokes (fingers would push the shadow into the camouflage).

eye shadow colour choice

the following guidelines illustrate how coloured eye shadows can affect the overall look and improve (or not improve) the eye colour. People will need to be reminded not to use a colour that would reintroduce any discolouration masked by their camouflage.

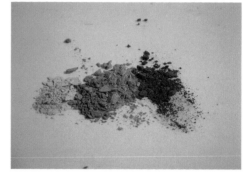

- brown, beige and cream are referred to as neutral colours, which work very well with a 'natural make-up' look and will be glamorous for all eye colours

- grey (light, medium or dark) is often regarded as an alternative to brown and is best used as an eyeliner, to create socket shadows or to blend with colours to make them tonal

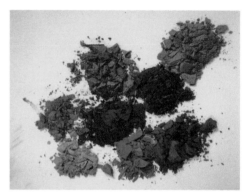

- pink, purple and red (these colours work well with greys) can look good on those with tanned skin and skin groups 4 to 6

- blue (pastel, vivid and dark): people may find it more flattering to blend these colours with a neutral or tonal shade, or to apply as an eyeliner

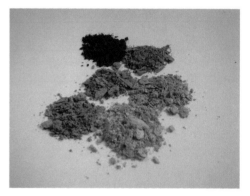

- green (pastel, vivid and dark), olive and yellow can look quite sludgy on tanned skin but can be a very effective method of camouflaging hyperpigmented skin to the eyelid without the need to use camouflage or concealer

- silver, gold, glitter and pearlised colours can add party glamour to the eyes but can emphasise fine lines, scar tissue and uneven skin texture

- black eye shadow can make an instant difference when applied carefully and can lift and reshape the eyes. It can also make eyes appear younger. A gentle, soft smudgy effect in this way will be glamorous to all age groups

counteracting pink eye

people who have a tinge of redness or pink either in the eyelid or surrounding the lashes (which seems to be more noticeable in winter) will find that applying a small amount of matt beige coloured eye shadow will make quite a drastic difference to the finished eye make-up. Avoid all shades of burgundy, purple, pink and any browns with red undertones.

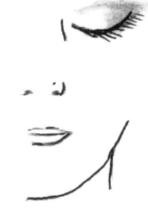

black eye shadow applied
at the temple corner

mascara

on no account should lines be drawn to resemble lashes (as was fashionable in the late 1960s). Where no lashes exist a soft, almost blurred, line usually achieves the best visual outcome.

product choice

mascara is available in many formats although people usually prefer those with an integral wand applicator. The wand and dispenser are designed to remove sufficient mascara for application – using a pumping action will not coat the wand with more product, but it will add air into the tube and cause oxidisation.

Waterproof mascara will need to be removed with cleansers designed for that purpose but is the best product to use for people whose eyes constantly tear or water. Whether someone prefers their mascara to contain fibres to lengthen the lashes, or just colour, is a matter of personal choice. Bushy black eyelashes look glamorous on youthful skins, but can be ageing to mature eyes. Mature people will benefit from dark brown or mid-brown mascara instead of black. If required, mascara can be applied over postiche lashes to combine them with the natural ones.

application technique

it is always best if people build up the density of mascara, allowing each application to dry before applying the next. The easiest method is to apply the wand to the base of the lashes and sweep up through the lashes to the tips. Make-up artists often use the wand at a 45° angle, which allows them to coat lashes individually from root to tip. When applying mascara on the lower lashes, people should use the wand carefully to apply a hint of colour rather than painting each individual lash, which can result in a "doll-like" appearance.

eyelash curlers

a gentle upward sweep to the lashes on the upper lid may not always be the natural growth and if lashes are short and straight, or grow at a right angle to the lid (or point downwards), then a shadow can be cast over the eye. Lashes can be curled to rectify lash shape. Some beauty salons offer eyelash perming (which should give a curl that lasts several weeks).

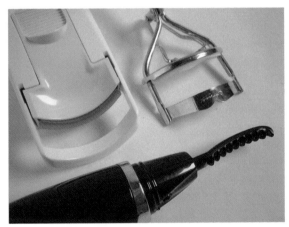

product choice

heated wand curlers will gently curl the lashes without clamping them and are less likely to break the hairs. Follow the manufacturer's instructions as some heated curlers can be used before mascara application, others recommend after.

03 manual and heated lash curlers

curling technique

eyelash curlers are best used in a two-stage process - to curl the lashes nearest to the roots then apply the curlers close to the tip of the lashes. This ensures the entire lashes are curled rather than just the roots. There is rarely a need to curl lashes under the eye.

eyeliner

is intended to cosmetically emphasise the eye shape and the product is applied as near to the root of the lashes as possible. Where no lashes exist, carefully outlining the eye will give the eye a frame and create a margin between the surrounding skin to the eyes. For those who have no lash hair, the long-term solution may be medical tattooing.

Black is probably the most popular shade. It can look very exotic on tanned skin and skin groups 3 to 6 but may be too harsh on skin groups 1 to 2 (where the use of slate grey, khaki green, dark blue or taupe brown is more flattering).

product choice

liners are available in various formats,

Pressed block will need to be moistened with clean water before use. Allow the product to dry thoroughly before capping and storage. An angled head brush can make application easier.

Liquid liners can flake off, which creates a very uneven look and can also be hazardous should flakes fall onto the eye or become trapped under contact lenses. Liquid liners are usually sold in a bottle with an integral applicator brush.

Although easy to apply, kohl pencils contain wax and are therefore liable to smudge. Liner pencils should be kept reasonably sharp using a pencil sharpener. As a hygienic precaution people will need to re-sharpen the liner between use.

Pen format liners may be the preferred choice of males and children because the packaging resembles a felt-tip pen. Pen liners are usually waterproof and longer lasting on the skin than other forms of liners. Care should be taken during application as these can often stain the skin – mistakes need to be removed quickly! The felt nib should be cleaned between use.

Waterproof liners may prove to be the better choice for those whose eyes water frequently, and will help prevent smudging should they inadvertently rub their eyes. However, they may cause an allergic reaction.

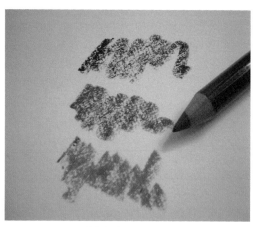

03 kohl pencils

application techniques for all products

care should be taken not to encircle the eye totally as this will make the eye appear smaller. Caution is needed when extending eyeliner past the eye shape, as a thin upward tick of liner at the temple corner can be mistaken for a wrinkle! People should be advised to avoid applying any products inside the rim of the eyelid as this can trigger allergic reactions and migrate under contact lenses; it can also make the eye appear smaller.

Avoid making the line the same thickness from start to finish as this will create a very round, startled eye shape. People may find it easier to start on the upper lid, drawing a thin tapered line from nose end to temple end of lid. From the middle of the eye, the line can become slightly thicker towards the finish at the end of the lashes. A line under the eye is applied in the same way.

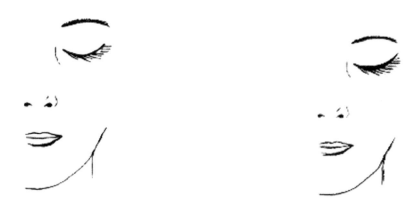

before liner   *graduated eyeliner applied to upper lash line*

blusher and contouring

blusher is used to give a healthy glow to cheeks; while some face shapes benefit from this, others do not! Blusher does not suit everyone and works best on those with natural well-defined cheekbones.

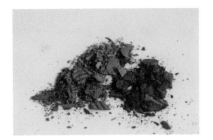

03 blusher colours

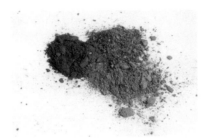

03 contour colours

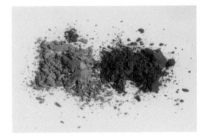

03 terracotta colours

Contouring gives shape to the face and accentuates cheekbones for those with a fuller face. The colour will need to be placed slightly lower – half cheekbone and half cheek hollow.

Blusher and contour that is applied too far across the cheek towards the nose will 'cut the face in half'. Ideally the product should not be applied further than the centre of the iris and should sweep in a very gentle arc towards the hairline. Any colour, when applied only to the cheekbone directly under the eye, will give a "doll-like" face.

Less is always best! The wrong colour will bring back any dermatosis concealed by foundation and/or camouflage. Blue-pink-red in a blusher will unwittingly bring back erythema (including port wine stains). The same problem arises when there is too much brown in the product when, for example, chloasma has been camouflaged. Pink blushers can bring back 'pink eye' effect.

Whether for blush or contour, a terracotta colour generally works well on most skin groups (pale for groups 1 to 4 and dark on groups 5 to 6). Golden browns can look glamorous on (faux) sun-tanned skin and will always give a healthy glow to skin groups 3 to 6. Avoid dark coloured bronzes on skin groups 1 to 2 as it can make the face look dirty.

product choice

blusher is usually sold in pressed powder format but can also be purchased as a loose powder – either product works well over camouflage. Blushers in liquid, gel and crème formats work best on skin that has no camouflage applied.

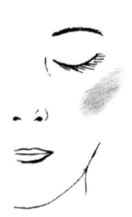

blusher placement

application technique

the brush needs to be firm, have compact hair and a large round head. If the brush hairs are too soft or too long, it will give no direction to movements. Square shaped brushes produce a stripe or even a delicately placed triangle. The accompanying brush that is often found in the packaging is usually square, flat and too small. Using this applicator will produce a stripe of colour which will distort the face shape.

Advise the person to wipe the brush over the product and gently tap off (never blow away) any excess. Lightly sweep the brush over the whole required area. If too much product is applied then the colour can be reduced by carefully rolling the foundation sponge or powder puff over the area. The same action will blend the blusher-contour and avoid any hard and unattractive margins.

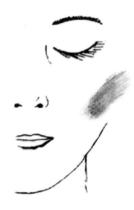

contour placement

lipstick

is a product that needs careful consideration. The colour used should make the lips look attractive and not draw attention to any fine lines around the mouth, scarring or distortion to lip shape. Depending on the shade chosen, lipstick can brighten a face. It can also have the opposite effect, making people look pale and tired. Lipstick can be applied over a lip stain and also very carefully over set camouflage. For people who have partial or no lips, the long-term solution may be medical tattooing.

product choice

crème camouflage products can be used to good effect as lipsticks – however, they will need sealing with powder or lipstick sealer.

Lipstick sealers are available, usually sold as a clear liquid which is painted over the lips once the lipstick (or camouflage product) has been applied. The sealer normally takes a few minutes to dry during which time the lips should remain motionless.

Long-lasting lipsticks and lip stains may be the solution for those who have excess saliva which can dribble over the lips.

Lipstick is usually sold in bullet shaped containers, but can be available as a crème in a pot, in pencil or pen format, or in a liquid formulation with an integral application brush.

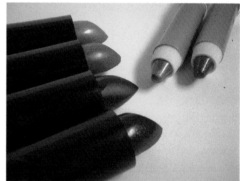

Lipstick is available in matt, semi-gloss, gloss, pearlised and sparkle finishes. Product colour and finish choice is individual. The following guidelines will help you understand which to advise:

- natural and pastel colours should make lips appear more full and should draw less attention to a distorted mouth shape

03 traditional lipstick bullets

- vivid and dark colours usually make lips appear smaller but at the same time will draw attention to the mouth area
- pearlised and lip-gloss will make small lips appear bigger – but will also emphasise any fine lines around the mouth
- matt and semi-gloss lipsticks suit all shapes and ages

  Lipstick may have undertones of blue or yellow, which will need to be taken into account when choosing a colour
- lipstick with blue undertones can emphasise comedones, rosacea, erythema, the 'pink eye' effect and melasma. However, lipsticks with blue undertones can make ivory teeth appear white and should counteract any sallowness in the complexion
- lipstick with yellow undertones can often flatter the skin's natural colour but may emphasise any sallowness to the skin and yellow staining on teeth.

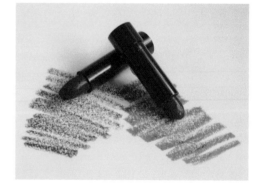

03 blue-red (left) and yellow-red (right) undertone to lipsticks

application technique

application is identical to that discussed in page 89 with obvious care not to dislodge any underlying camouflage.

People may wish to use a pencil after the lip colour: the lubricant of the lipstick means the two blend together and create a softer, more natural finish. This has the added benefit of producing a barrier, which prevents the margin of the lipstick bleeding into the skin around the mouth. As a hygiene precaution, re-sharpen the lip pencil between each use.

the important role of skin camouflage: peoples' experiences and case histories

"I can save your life, but you have to live it"

published by kind permission from Christine Piff, Let's Face It

I'm fuming!   With the ongoing campaign to raise public awareness for those coping with visual differences, I would like to tell of an incident experienced by my daughter when she took her three year old son for his first swimming lesson at the local leisure centre.

To put you in the picture my three year old grandson has a full birthmark running from his right elbow down to his right thumb. It was not apparent when he was born but emerged over the following ten days after he was born. At first it was a very vivid total scarlet mark that resembled a severe burn and was very prominent against his very pale colouring. It has been monitored regularly and it started to break down when he was about eighteen months old. It is now regarded as a salmon flash, is much paler in colour and the consultant advises that it will probably have disappeared by the time he is seven years old.

He began his first series of swimming lessons at our local leisure centre four weeks ago and is progressing very well. However, an incident that took place last week left me so shocked and appalled that I felt it needed to be reported to BASC as well as the relevant people at the centre.

On climbing out of the pool one of the swimming instructors noticed his arm and enquired as to what the mark was. My grandson said it was a special mark (remember he is only three and this is one of the answers that he can remember when asked by curious children at nursery). By this time my daughter arrived at the poolside and had overheard the question and the following conversation took place between the swimming instructor and my daughter:

Daughter*: "It is a birthmark"*

Swimming Instructor: *"I have never seen a birthmark like that"*

Daughter*: "It's called a salmon flash"*

Swimming Instructor: *"It doesn't look like a birthmark to me and I don't think he should be in the water with other children................"*

This conversation took place in front of the other mothers and children at the poolside and, because my daughter did not want to take issue with the swimming instructor in front of her son, plus the fact that she was also seething with anger, she walked away deciding to deal with the situation later.

However, when turning to leave the pool my daughter overheard the swimming instructor saying to her colleague that she *"didn't think it looked like a birthmark but more of a skin disease and it made her feel sick to look at it".*

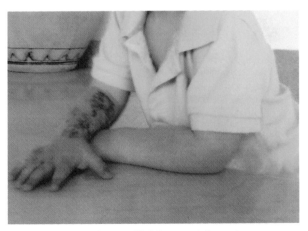

grandson with his special mark
© BASC member 2049

Well, I am sure your reaction would have been the same as mine – total disbelief at the ignorance, rudeness and lack of sensitivity on the part of the instructor.

Needless to say my daughter and husband subsequently sought an appointment with the manager of the leisure centre and the matter is in hand. However, as an irate 'gran'ma' I would like this published so that other children do not experience the same appalling treatment. Fortunately my grandson was not fazed by the incident – he is used to children asking about his arm, but it beggars belief that an adult in a teaching and training position with children should behave in such an appalling manner.

BASC Member 2049

Skin camouflage has been the biggest single influence on my life.

It has opened many doors, allowing me to lead a completely normal and fulfilling life. Low self-esteem, a total lack of confidence and a continuous fear of drawing attention to myself were all features of my personality before I discovered the existence of the camouflage which has totally changed my life. The products are so effective in concealing my extensive facial port wine stain that many people I know have no idea of its existence.

I now feel a very different person and have totally changed from a quiet, withdrawn person into that of a confident, out going and lively woman. My working life, thanks to the success of the camouflage, has been very much in the public eye. I worked as an air stewardess for a major airline, I have performed as a professional dancer and now I am currently the Head of Dance at a large comprehensive school. All of these professions were only distant dreams to me before I discovered the 'life-saving' properties of skin camouflage.

After 30 years of wearing my camouflage so successfully, I am now married with a beautiful son and have established myself as a highly successful teacher within my Educational career. None of this would ever have been possible had I not discovered camouflage which helped me to overcome my fears and restrictions of living with a birthmark.

Rosalyn Mawazini

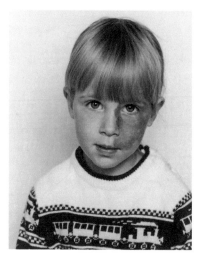

as a very shy child
© Mrs Rosalyn Mawazini

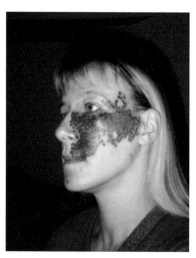

post laser surgery
© Mrs Rosalyn Mawazini

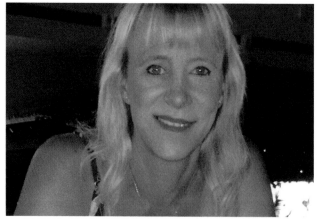

me, 2014
© Mrs Rosalyn Mawazini

Having a scar means never having a day off I sustained burns to my face, body and hands in an acid attack. I remember looking at my face in the mirror for the first time in hospital. My psychologist was with me. My scars looked so much worse than I had imagined. Whenever I left the burns unit to go to appointments elsewhere in the hospital people turned and stared at me, looking shocked. During this time I felt sorry for them because they had to look at me. I could sense that people felt nervous around me. After I was discharged home I remember going shopping with my mum. I wore a wide-brimmed hat, sunglasses and scarf. In one awful incident a shopping assistant pulled off my hat, looked at my face with a disgusted expression and shouted at me to get out of the shop. That was an extreme example, but milder reactions from strangers were no easier to cope with.

The first time I went out with my sister to a shopping centre I felt like I wanted to disappear when I noticed groups of boys nudging each other, whispering and pointing. During that shopping trip I tried to go to the make-up counters but I found the assistants too intimidating and my sister had to shop for me. People would often ask me what had happened, or make a comment on my appearance. Although they were usually well meaning, it actually made me feel worse. I couldn't understand why people felt they could stare or comment on how I looked, as if having scars made me public property.

Now I would tell someone in the same situation that most of the time those people are not intentionally cruel, they're uneducated and they're seeing something they aren't used to seeing because there isn't enough awareness. However I think it's important for people to realise that one look to satisfy your own curiosity, or one misguided question or comment could be enough to tip someone over the edge that day and stop them from doing things like leaving the house or going back to work. Regaining my confidence again was a long, slow process, but little things helped me along the way. I remember my parents throwing a party for me at home; it was the first time I'd seen all my friends and I was so relieved when they didn't turn away in disgust, but ran over and gave me a hug. My brother arranged for me to meet another burns survivor who had sustained burns ten years before; I didn't believe that I'd ever look as good as her but it gave me hope that one day my scars would be paler and less shocking. I remember taking a night off from wearing my pressure mask (which I had to wear for 2 years to flatten my scars) and getting dressed up to go to a party in a bar; for the first time I started to feel a bit more like myself.

I still have bad days when I feel unconfident, but when I do, I tell myself that it's normal because everyone has bad days! Camouflage and make-up products have been a useful tool for me at different stages of my recovery. When I stopped wearing the mask I experimented with different kinds of camouflage and regular makeup brands. While I was an inpatient I saw a skin camouflage practitioner; I built up my hopes that I would look much better afterwards, but because the skin on my face wasn't healed she could only put some product on the scars on my hand. With hindsight it would have been better to have waited as this session only made

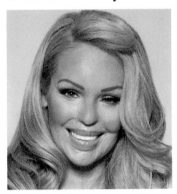

Katie Piper – over the counter make-up used © Michael Fasani

me feel worse! After I was discharged I went to a camouflage consultation in a beauty salon. I felt very nervous but I was desperate for something to improve my appearance. Afterwards I was disappointed because you could see the texture of my scars, I didn't realise then that the camouflage would only help to make the colour even; but I was proud that I had gone through with the appointment and it gave me some hope that I could look different in the future.

I think the big turning point in my life was the decision to help others. At the big launch party for my charity I chose not to wear camouflage; this was partly because I didn't want to hide my scars. These days sometimes I choose to wear make-up over the scars on my face, neck and chest and sometimes I go without; it just depends on how I'm feeling and what I'm doing that day. I always wear over-the-counter make up for TV work and then it's nice when I'm doing my other jobs and relaxing to go make-up free and enjoy the extra time eating breakfast! I find it helps me just to know I have the choice.

**Katie Piper
founder of the Katie Piper Foundation**

founded in 2009, KPF is dedicated to improving the delivery of burns rehabilitation and scar management. The Foundation helps people with burns and scars throughout their recovery and on an on-going basis. Our vision is a world where scars do not limit a person's function, social inclusion or sense of well-being. More information can be found at www.katiepiperfoundation.org.uk

skin camouflage helps people with facial scarring say "I Do!" once more

A wedding wouldn't be complete without wedding photos to immortalize the happy occasion. In Taiwan, bridal photography is a big affair and is one of the most important steps in wedding preparations. Brides usually cannot wait to get their stylized and glamorized photographs taken, which involves many changes of dresses to show the bride at her most beautiful. However, for people with facial scarring this process is sometimes fraught with distress. Some people of Sunshine Foundation said that they didn't feel beautiful during their wedding, so they didn't take any pictures and lack a memento of their happy day.

To compensate for this the Sunshine Foundation organized, with the help of students from the Department of *Cosmetic* Science at Chang-Gung University, a special activity that allowed people to shoot the bridal photos of their dream. Thanks to skin camouflage techniques, as well as styling by professional bridal photographers, five couples were able to go back to the time when they said "I do!" and create new memories.

For some of the couples, it was the first time to wear wedding clothes and pose for pictures, so they were quite nervous. But thanks to the encouragement of Sunshine staff and student volunteers, they started to feel comfortable in front of the camera and enjoy this special experience, smiling and striking poses like movie stars.

Hui-Li and A-Chung were one of these couples. Hui-Li was burned over 80% of her body when she was young. Many years later, she met A-Chung who saw past her scars and appreciated her petulant personality. They married but never had the chance to immortalize the event in photos, so they were eager to take part in this activity. Hui-Li and A-Chung thoroughly enjoyed themselves, posing in front of the camera for serious romantic shots and more playful ones. The love between them radiates through the pictures and Hui-Li said: "Now we have beautiful wedding pictures to immortalize our love!"

Sunshine Foundation has been providing skin camouflage services since training with BASC in 2002 and offer individual and group consultations to people with facial scarring as well as training volunteers to ensure that this service is available across Taiwan. Skin camouflage is also often used during various activities that encourage psychological rehabilitation and social participation of people with facial scars - these activities help and enhance public understanding.

Esther LIEN,
Skin Camouflage Service Planner, Sunshine Social Welfare Foundation

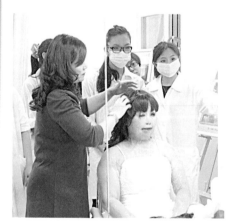

during the camouflage
and make-up session
© *Sunshine Social Welfare Foundation*

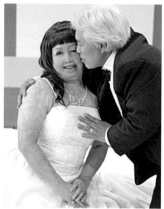

delighted bride
© *Sunshine Social Welfare*
Foundation

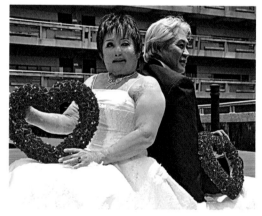

bride and groom
© *Sunshine Social Welfare Foundation*

Sunshine Social Welfare Foundation is a nonprofit organization based in Taiwan and established in 1981 to provide comprehensive services to burn survivors and people with facial disfigurement, to assist them in their physical, psychological and social rehabilitation; to uphold their human rights and dignity.

Life without hair Your hair is your identity, your sensuality, sexuality and how you present yourself to the world. We are bombarded daily on how we should curl, straighten, colour, wash and style our hair. Hair is the first thing you notice on someone, just before you look at their face and body. You judge people by their grooming, their style, their amount of product and colouring.

Image if you started to loose patches and/or completely loose all your hair. How would that make you feel when you looked in the mirror? Will your partner find you attractive anymore? Will people think you are sick?

In alopecia areata, multifactorial triggers are cited from inflammatory stress response, genetic, autoimmune responses, immunisation, environmental and diet as the cause. The scientific community continues to investigate but funding into research is poor. So what do you do in the meantime when dealing with emotional distress of an altered body image that impacts on your personal, social and work life?

Your ability to cope depends on your coping mechanisms and social support network. For people who struggle will find themselves at a higher risk of depression, social phobia and anxiety disorders. If left unchecked it can and does affect people's jobs and relationships. Therefore, there is a real need for greater awareness of alopecia and the devastation it can bring, as well as to challenge societal norms.

Hairpieces, wigs and hair integrated systems, head scarves, semi-permanent make-up to recreate eyebrows, or choosing not to wear anything are all effective ways to cope psychologically. For those who choose to wear hair systems there can then be an underlying fear of being discovered and altered perceptions of self 'am I me when I wear my wig? who am I when I take it off?'

It depends on a person's emotional state and how they are able to adapt to their new body image and self-identity. It's also influenced by personal budget, as wigs range in price, depending on the type of synthetic wig and the quality and ethical sourcing of human hair. Choices might be further limited depending on the provision funded by your Clinical Commission Group. Individuals can find peer support at Alopecia UK and the answers to many practical questions.

Promoting a positive body image is fundamental when advising individuals that hair loss will not stop them from achieving their personal or work goals or prevent them from having successful relationships. It is also important to reassure, it might seem impossible at first, that they can become confident and deal with their appearance.

Jackie Tomlinson

Chair of Trustee's Alopecia UK

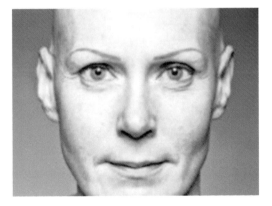

Jackie Tomlinson
© Daniel Regan

founded in 2005, Alopecia UK provides impartial information, advice and support to those affected by hair loss. They raise awareness to the general public and healthcare professionals about alopecia and its psychological impact.

I never expected to develop rosacea at the age of 58! I'd had the odd occasional spot as a teenager (don't we all?) so it came as a shock to find that my cheeks, nose and chin were getting redder every day – and that within a short space of time I had lots of spots too!

My GP sent me to see the dermatologist, who simply said "rosacea" and prescribed a medicated ointment to control the spots. The ointment seemed to encourage, rather than discourage, outbreaks, so I went back to the GP. The GP re-referred me to the dermatology out patients department, and this time I was prescribed oral antibiotics to control the spots.

The tablets worked, although I did get the occasion "blind spot" (I think this is called a papule) which were very painful and itchy. I would have rest periods between courses of tablets, and during the rest the spots would reappear. I tried not to "squeeze" the spots – but it's difficult as you think it will clear up quicker if you do this…always careful to wrap clean fingers in tissue, and to be as hygienic as possible.

Then, at an annual medical check, it was discovered I had high blood pressure and needed a daily pill to manage that. I was advised that the antibiotic and blood pressure pills would not be compatible. The choice would seem to be live longer with spots, or risk a stroke/heart attack but have spot free skin. Naturally I chose the former option!

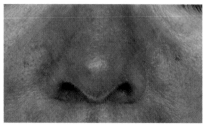

rosacea
© BASC member 1002

The dermatologist mentioned skin camouflage, so I thought I might as well give it a try. It hasn't affected the spots – they still come and go at their own will – but it does help cover the redness to my nose, cheeks, chin and forehead. I can usually get away with a heavy duty make-up foundation during the summer, when my skin is warmer….but come the cold-damp weather I need to apply just a bit of camouflage to reduce the "purple" shadow that comes through a make-up foundation.

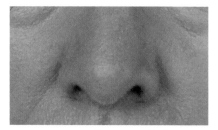

camouflage applied
© BASC member 1002

Ten years on and I've resigned myself to "teenage acne skin" with permanent blushing! As yet I've not developed any thread veins, nor has the skin become thicker on my nose – but maybe this will be just a matter of time!

Who'd have thought that I would need camouflage at my age…..and for a medical condition I though could be better controlled, or perhaps rare in my age group. Reading Dr Google, apparently it's common!

Why should I be expected to discuss my medical history with strangers? People are curious and make assumptions. To satisfy both nosy reactions they often ask me "have you been burnt?" Others grimace and bluntly ask "is it catching?" I don't challenge them about their image – so why should they do so to me?

I've had psoriasis for half my life; I am happily married, have a wonderful daughter, son-in-law and granddaughter. Like my friends, they are unconcerned about my skin and basically so am I. I agree it is an inconvenience, and yes I would prefer to have flawless skin but as it's a chronic condition I have learnt to live with it and not for it. But, to be honest it's "the others" who do make life tedious!

I accept it must be very difficult for someone who has just developed a skin condition to adjust and go about their life when people can be so (mainly unintentionally) cruel. I can understand why it is easier not to make

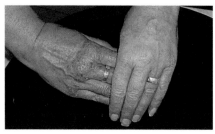

psoriasis - right hand without, left hand with camouflage applied
© BASC

eye contact in the belief that "if I didn't see them, then they wont see me!" Not wishing to sound paranoiac, you do develop a sixth sense, and you do begin to realise that people are avoiding making contact with you – I must be one of the few who welcome self service check-outs! You hear the whispers and sniggers; so I wear my camouflage when the mood suits me – to blend in with everyone else and not stand out in the crowd – that way I am less likely to be challenged and expected to respond to someone asking about my medical history when I am just out and about, like them.

Elizabeth Allen

a *"potted history" of skin camouflage*

*if you want something enough, then tell everyone you meet about it
and in the end you will find someone who will help you achieve it.*

Joyce Allsworth (1985)

a "potted" history of Skin Camouflage

In response to questions often asked, and to link with pride the history of BASC, here is an outline of the gradual evolution of skin camouflage, including Joyce Allsworth's inspirational role. Joyce instigated the camouflage service within the British Red Cross and founded The British Association of Skin Camouflage. She also wrote and published in 1985 *Skin Camouflage – A Guide to Remedial Techniques* (now out of print).

The history of wearing skin camouflage products has been concealed by the passage of time; most records are lost and, sadly, a lot of information relies more on rumour and hearsay than fact. However certain dates and names are available from archive sources and from those we can begin to create a picture of events.

Before any product became available there had to be a cause – a reason that made wearing cosmetics (and camouflage) socially accepted and marketed. We know that throughout the history of cosmetics, wearing make-up had always been considered the prerogative of the rich, as well as having an association with those involved in the performing arts and prostitution. Those who wore any form of artifice had to make their own products or have a servant to do that menial task for them. During the late 18th century opinions changed. No longer did the rich wear obvious make-up, and the wearing of any cosmetic morphed to be a social sign of falsehood, a vanity that did not equate with good and god-fearing behaviour. From the numerous social and political upheavals of the 19th and 20th centuries we can begin to appreciate the causes that permitted use of make-up and skin camouflage to become socially acceptable. Once the social climate had changed, manufacturers began to produce an array of products. Today the cosmetics and toiletries industries show annual multi-billion dollar sales.

The women's suffrage movement (which gained momentum from the middle of the 19th century) not only resulted in women having a political voice and the opportunities of better education and employment, emancipation also gave them choices – one was to wear make-up without encountering social discrimination. In New York, during the early years of the 20th century, the women marching in support of the female textile workers' strike wore bright red lipstick. Interestingly, Elizabeth Arden joined the march, even though most of the strikers would not have had the means to afford most cosmetics on sale at that time.

During the same timeframe, at the other side of America, another movement was affecting society's perception of beauty. The cause of this massive interest in cosmetics was the invention of the film industry. The popularity of the cinema did much to promote a flawless complexion – and ushered in an era in which women would also want to look like their screen idol. The 'beauty business' had begun! Because of the intense lighting required during filming, there was a need to create make-up that would withstand the performer's perspiration. Undoubtedly in those pioneering days the main contributor to perfecting such durable make-up was Max Factor. Maksymilian Faktorowicz Americanised his name to Max Faktor (1877-1938) emigrated from Poland to the USA in 1902, and it was then that a spelling error occurred in his surname. Factor moved to California in 1908–9 and had, by 1914, perfected a flexible greasepaint make-up suitable for those early filming requirements. His other major make-up innovations, especially pan-cake (Academy Award 1928), without which it would have been impossible to take full advantage of the light and shade sensitivity of Panchromatic film, led the way for natural looking film, television and street make-up. For decades he was the un-crowned king of Hollywood and his make-up became an international leading brand. His concealer, pan-stick and pan-cake cosmetics are still sold today.

In 1918 Max Factor created the 'colour harmony' principle, in which all products were harmonised to tone with the wearer's natural skin, eye and hair colour. It was the first time in cosmetic history that powder, rouge, eye make-up and lipstick were co-ordinated to suit blue-eyed blondes, brown-eyed brunettes and so on. Because audiences wanted the same cosmetic look as their screen idol, Factor launched his cosmetics for general sale in 1927 – his brand advertisements were the first to use celebrities to endorse the products. As a wigmaker, Factor also perfected human hair wigs and false eyelashes for the film industry, which, in turn, filtered their way onto general sale. He also worked with American plastic surgeons after World War I to create a cosmetic suitable for use as skin camouflage – performers having scars and dermatoses that needed concealing too – but mainly for veterans who had been severely burnt.

In 1928 an American university graduate, Lydia O'Leary, utilised her knowledge of chemistry and love of painting to develop a make-up foundation that would conceal her facial port wine stain. Her product, Covermark®, became the first foundation to receive a patent by the US Patent & Trademark Office and paved the way for camouflage products to become accepted as a medical aid, rather than a beauty product. Her original formula was a thick liquid, which later became the camouflage crème we know today. Interestingly it was estimated in 1928 that approximately 15% of sales were to men.

Max Factor died in 1938, the same year that his company was requested by the Ministry of Defence to formulate shades of pan-cake make-up for commandos to use as camouflage during World War II (for example, 'jungle green'). At the same time the qualities in the product were recognised by the medical profession to use as skin camouflage to mask injuries, so his Factor Company began to create colours suitable for street, as well as theatrical wear.

World War I and World War II led to acceleration in advances in medical techniques. Survival from horrific injury became more achievable and plastic surgeons tested new procedures that would, later in the century, transform both the medical and beauty professions.

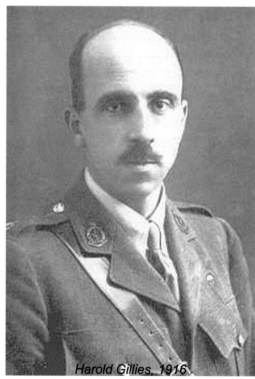

Harold Gillies, 1916
photograph in public domain

Although only 32 years old when World War I began, Major Harold Delf Gillies (FRCS RAMC) pressured the Ministry of Defence to open a centre (Queens Hospital, Sidcup, Kent) to develop plastic surgery techniques to repair facial injuries. He performed thousands of pioneering operations there, and was considered by his patients to be the hero of the Somme. In 1920 Dr Gillies published *Plastic Surgery for the Face*, and was later knighted in recognition of his work. Sir Harold was instrumental in founding the British Association of Plastic Surgeons (BAPS) and was its First President; 36 people attended the first meeting, which was held on 20th November 1946 at the Royal College of Surgeons, London. In 2006 BAPS changed their name to British Association of Plastic, Reconstructive and Aesthetic Surgeons (BAPRAS).

New Zealand-born Gillies (1882-1960) persuaded his cousin to forsake general for plastic surgery. Archibald McIndoe (1900–1960), also born in New Zealand, came to the UK in 1930, taking up an appointment as clinical assistant in the Department of Plastic Surgery at St Bartholomew's Hospital, London. In 1938 he was appointed consultant to the RAF and, when war broke out in 1939, he selected the newly built Queen Victoria Hospital at East Grinstead as his base. Sir Archibald McIndoe was also involved with the forming of BAPS and was its third president. He was knighted in 1947.

Sir Archibald pioneered saline baths (for burn injuries) during his work at the Queen Victoria Hospital. However, Sir Archibald knew that his patients also needed to regain their self-esteem to enjoy a happy and fulfilled life. His philosophy was that treatment should always be 50% medical and 50% psychological. He allowed his patients to wear their uniforms and civilian clothing (rather than pyjamas) and gave them the liberty to go outside the hospital whenever they wished to local dance halls and public houses.

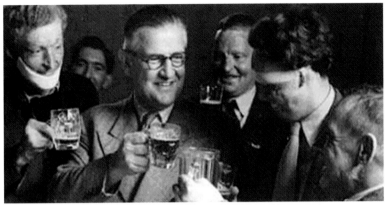

Archibald McIndoe with members of the Guinea Pig Club
© the Guinea Pig Club

McIndoe realised that his patients could help each other by mutual support; in 1942, with 28 founder members (there were 649 by the end of the war), the first patients' support group (run by patients for patients) was born. They called themselves 'the Guinea Pig Club' as much of their surgery was experimental. McIndoe described it as the most exclusive club in the world, adding that the entrance fee was something most men would not pay. He also appreciated that to help them with reintegration, his guinea pigs might also benefit from a durable skin coloured preparation – skin camouflage! Whether Sir Archibald had seen samples of Covermark remains uncertain, but he was familiar with Max Factor's pan-cake.

Eve Gardiner (1916-1992) worked in close association with Sir Archibald and Sir Harold Gillies during World War II when the Max Factor Salon in Bond Street, London also offered their services for war victims. Eve is probably best remembered for her remarkable work in teaching those who are partially sighted and blind to apply make-up; she later instigated a training programme with the British Red Cross for them to provide that service. We know that Eve and Joyce Allsworth were colleagues, although when their friendship began is not documented.

Records suggest that Sir Archibald also contacted his friend Thomas Blake (an analytic chemist) to create a topical crème that was skin coloured to help conceal burn scar tissue. Thomas Blake set about this task, perfecting Veil Cover Cream, which was first used by the Guinea Pigs at East Grinstead and eventually went on general sale in 1952. Thomas Blake initially created just three skin tone colours (Natural was shortly followed by Medium and then the misnomer Dark – because it was darker than the other two). Later, Joyce Allsworth was very instrumental in helping Veil develop new colours. Brown and Yellow were her ideas and she also helped by suggesting other skin tones and complementary colours. Thomas Blake died in 1979.

Elizabeth Arden also knew Harold Gillies and, during World War II, created a crème to help conceal. Known as 'scar cream', she toured hospitals throughout the USA in the post-war years (children's wards in particular) promoting her products. Elizabeth Arden was invited during World War II to create a morale-boosting make-up kit for the American Marine Corps Women's Reserve. She was thrilled to observe them drilling at Camp Wilmington, North Carolina – all wearing her red lipstick, rouge and nail polish that matched their uniform's chevrons. Cosmetics manufacturers were quick to realise that camouflage products have a rightful place in their ranges and most, if not all, now sell concealers.

At the time of printing, The British National Health Service lists brands of camouflage within the *Monthly Index of Medical Specialities* (Borderline Substances) and the *British National Formulary* for reimbursement on form FP10 (which means they can be obtained on prescription at doctor's discretion). These are Covermark, Veil, Keromask (originally developed during the late 1950s by Innoxa USA to camouflage port wine stains, and recognised by the British Medical Association shortly afterwards) and the leading German brand Dermacolor (devised by Kryolan during the 1960s). Dermablend (which was formulated by American dermatologist Dr Craig Roberts in 1983) was available on prescription until 2005. Additional to the above, other products that are included on the *Chemical & Drug Price List* can be obtained via a doctor's hand written prescription.

In the late 1950s a cosmetics company called Atkinsons realised that skin care products could do much to improve the morale of hospital patients. An experimental scheme was set up at St Clement's Hospital in the East End of London; it proved so successful that in 1959 the British Red Cross was then asked to take over from the nurses trained by Atkinsons and organise a Beauty Care Service in hospitals throughout Great Britain. Joyce Allsworth became an instructor for this service, which was directed in London by Ruth Russell. By 1977 the Red Cross had celebrated training its 3,000th beauty care volunteer.

Another pioneer was Doreen Trust – born with a facial birthmark – who founded the Disfigurement Guidance Centre. She did much to promote camouflage, writing papers for *The British Journal of Dermatology* and publishing *Skin Deep, An Introduction to Skin Camouflage and Disfigurement Therapy* (Paul Harris 1977). Doreen Trust remains energetic in promoting LASER treatments, especially for port wine stains.

Joyce Allsworth was serving with the WAAF at North Weald, Essex during World War II and was shocked by the facial burns of one particular airman. She came to realise that it was not enough to feel empathy but that something more should be done to help burn survivors. Records suggest that Joyce was aware of the pioneering work by Sir Harold Gillies, Sir Archibald McIndoe and Thomas Blake although no documentation exists of their first interaction. She studied beauty therapy and theatrical make-up artistry skills at the London School of Fashion, but it was not until the Stockport air disaster (1967) that Joyce transferred her skills to concentrate exclusively on skin camouflage techniques.

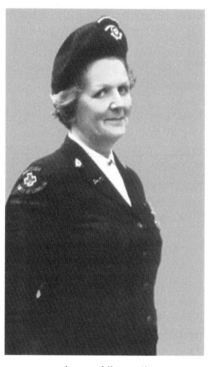

Joyce Allsworth

At the request of Mr J S P Wilson (consultant plastic surgeon at St George's Hospital, London) Joyce opened an outpatient clinic to help people who would benefit from skin camouflage. Joyce, who at that time was the chief trainer and examiner for the Red Cross London Beauty Care Service, began to lobby politicians, medical professionals, and indeed anyone she thought might help her promote a skin camouflage service within the Red Cross.

In 1975 the Department of Health and Social Services carried out a survey which found that dermatologists were anxious to have this specialised provision in their hospitals. The DHSS approached the British Red Cross Society offering to assist with funding for a training programme to provide a skin camouflage service. A meeting was organised; Ruth Russell and Joyce Allsworth were invited to attend. Joyce's dreams were at long last being fulfilled when (with an initial DHSS grant of £1,500) she instigated the training programme at the Society's training centre at Barnett Hill, Surrey. Within three years she had trained 90 students who were providing a Red Cross camouflage service in approximately 50 locations within Great Britain. Joyce continued to train Red Cross skin camouflage practitioners for the following eight years until she left the service.

It occurred to Joyce that National Health Service skin camouflage provision excluded those who attended private clinics, and those who did not wish to get their doctor involved for fear of being accused of vanity. She also realised that a textbook was needed to encourage people to learn the skills of skin camouflage, either for their own personal use or for use on others. Founded in 1985 BASC is the direct result of a request to form a national support association for skin camouflage professionals through which the principles, skills, expertise and new techniques could be shared - and the rest, as they say, is history! In order to protect its members from financial liability, BASC became a Company Limited by Guarantee in 2007 and in 2008 BASC became a Charity registered in England and Wales.

When Joyce died in 1994 she had devoted over 50 years to promoting skin camouflage and training practitioners. Thanks to her tireless work, skin camouflage is no longer a service that has to be hidden away! The British Association of Skin Camouflage proudly continues the pioneering work of Joyce Allsworth and the other pioneers and innovators who made such critical contributions during the 20th century.

Now, in the 21st century, BASC is at the leading edge of skin camouflage, drawing on its rich history and experience, to continually look at ways of perfecting techniques and services for people whilst motivating and encouraging health professionals and other practitioners to become involved with skin camouflage.

BASC trained practitioners pride themselves on the principles and arts they practice
- the skill of skin camouflage application -
and their role in helping others to
face the world, with confidence

directory of useful organisations website links

recommended reading

cosmetic ingredients common to camouflage products

index

directory of useful organisations website links

all addresses were correct at the time of inclusion; the British Association of Skin Camouflage apologise, but cannot accept responsibility for any inconvenience caused by changes to name and contact details.

medical and surgical consultants belong to a number of recognised associations that demand a high level of training; these associations provide lists of their registered practitioners for other professionals or the general public to check against

Association of the British Pharmaceutical Industry	www.abpi.org.uk
British Association of Aesthetic Plastic Surgeons	www.baaps.org.uk
British Association of Cosmetic Doctors	www.cosmeticdoctors.co.uk
British Association of Dermatologists	www.bad.org.uk
British Association of Oral and Maxillofacial Surgeons	www.baoms.org.uk
British Association of Otorhinolaryngologists	www.entuk.org
British Association of Plastic, Reconstructive and	www.bapras.org.uk

Aesthetic Surgeons (formerly known as BAPS, the British Association of Plastic Surgeons)

British Association of MR Radiographers	www.bamrr.org
British Association of Sclerotherapists	www.basclerotherapy.com
British Dental Association	www.bda.org
British Dermatological Nursing Group	www.bdgn.org.uk
British Oculoplastic Surgery Society	ww.bopss.co.uk
British Skin Foundation	www.britishskinfoundation.org.uk
Cancer Networks	www.db.gov.uk
College of Occupational Therapists	www.cot.co.uk
Dermatology Skin Information Site	www.dermatology.co.uk
Electronic Medicines Compendium	www.medicines.org.uk
European Academy of Dermatology and Venereology	www.eadv.org
European Association of Plastic Surgeons	www.euraps.org
Genetic Interest Group	www.gig.org.uk
Institute of Maxillofacial Prosthetists & Technologists	www.impt.org
International Society of Aesthetic Plastic Surgeons	www.isaps.org
Medical Pages – the UK health portal	www.medicalpages.co.uk
National Institute for Health & Clinical Excellence	www.nice.org.uk
National Library for Health	www.library.nhs.uk/skin
(skin conditions specialist library)	
National Voices	www.nationalvoices.org.uk
NHS direct	www.nhsdirect.nhs.uk
NHS-Primary Care Trusts	www.nhs.uk
Patients' Information Site	www.patient.co.uk
Primary Care Dermatology Society	www.pcds.org.uk
Royal College of Nursing	www.rcn.org.uk
Royal College of Surgeons	www.rcseng.ac.uk
Royal Pharmaceutical Society of GB	www.rpsgb.org.uk
Society of Vascular Technology	www.svtgbi.org.uk

Surgical Dressing Manufacturers Association	www.sdma.org.uk
Tissue Viability Society	www.tvs.org.uk
Wound Care Society	www.woundcaresociety.org

American Academy of Dermatology	www.aad.org
American Academy of Facial Plastic and Reconstructive Surgery	www.aafprs.org
American Society for Aesthetic Plastic Surgery	www.surgery.org
American Society for Dermatologic Surgery	www.asda-net.org
American Society of Plastic Surgeons	www.plasticsurgery.org
American Vitiligo Research Foundation	www.avrf.org

British Association of Beauty Therapy and Cosmetology	www.babtac.com
British Institute & Association of Electrolysists	www.electrolysis.co.uk
Federation of Holistic Therapists	www.fht.org.uk
Guild of Professional Beauty Therapists	www.beautyguild.com
Hairdressing and Beauty Industry Authority	www.habia.org
Institute of Trichologists	www.trichologists.org.uk
International Federation of Aromatherapists	www.ifaroma.org
International Society of Professional Aromatherapists	www.ifaroma.org

Banbury Postiche	www.banburypostiche.co.uk
Clinique Laboratories Ltd	www.clinique.com
Dawn Cragg	www.downcragg.net
DermaGard (protection UV window film)	www.bonwyke.co.uk
Finishing Touches	www.wakeupwithmakeup.co.uk
Lynton Lasers	www.lynton.co.uk
Meda Pharmaceuticals (Dermatix)	www.dermatix.co.uk
My New Hair	www.mynewhair.org
Nouveau Contour	www.nouveaucontour.co.uk
SilDerm Scar Gel	www.cranagehealth.com
Sinclair (Kelo-Cote)	www.kelo-cote.co.uk
Ski:n@Lasercare	www.lasercareskinclinic.com
Smith & Nephew (CicaCare)	www.smith-nephew.com
SunSense (skin protection)	www.sunsense.co.uk
SunSibility (protective clothing)	www.sunsibility.co.uk
Ultrasun (skin protection)	www.ultrasun.co.uk

Aniquem	www.aniquem.org
(providing support to burn injured children, Peru)	
Sunshine Social Welfare Foundation, Taiwan	www.sunshine.org.tw
(providing services to burn survivors and people with scarring)	

Albinism Fellowship	www.albinism.org.uk
Allergy UK	www.allergyuk.org
Alopecia Awareness	www.alopecia-awareness.org.uk
Alopecia UK	www.alopecia.org.uk
Behcet's Syndrome Society	www.behcets.org.uk
Birthmark Support Group	www.birthmarksupportgroup.org.uk
Burn Support Groups,	www.burnsupportgroupdatabase.com
Organisation and Burn Camp database	
Burned Children's Club (Essex)	www.burnedchildrensclub.org.uk
Cancer BACUP	www.cancerbacup.org.uk
Cancer Research UK	www.cancerresearchuk.org
Changing Faces	www.changingfaces.org.uk
Children's Fire and Burn Trust	www.childrensfireandburntrust.org.uk
Cleft Lip and Palate Association	www.clapa.com
Congenital Melanocytic Naevus	www.caringmattersnow.co.uk
Counselling	www.counselling-directory.org.uk
Contact A Family	www.cafamily.org.uk
(for families with disabled children)	
Darier's Disease Support Group	www.dariers.com
DebRA : Epidermolysis Bullosa	www.debra.org.uk
Ectodermal Dysplasia Society	www.ectodermaldysplasia.org
Ehlers-Danlos Support Group	www.ehlers-danlos.org
Gorlin Syndrome Group	www.gorlingroup.co.uk
Herpes Viruses Association	www.hva.org.uk
Hyperhidrosis Support Group	www.hyperhidrosisuk.org
HITS - Hypomelanosis of Ito Syndrome	www.e-fervour.com
Ichthyosis Support Group	www.ichthyosis.org.uk
Katie Piper Foundation	www.katiepiperfoundation.org.uk
Latex Allergy Support Group	www.lasg.co.uk
LEPRA : the British Leprosy Relief Association	www.lepra.co.uk
Let's Face It	www.lets-face-it.org.uk
Long-term Medical Conditions Alliance	www.lmca.org.uk
Lupus UK	www.lupusuk.org.uk
Lymphoedema Support Network	www.lymphoedema.org
Lymphoma Association	www.lymphomas.org
Marfan Association UK	www.marfan-association.org.uk
Myositis Support Group	www.myositis.org.uk
National Eczema Society	www.eczema.org
National Lichen Sclerosus Group	www.lichensclerosus.org
National Self Harm Alliance	www.selfharmalliance.org
Neurofibromatosis Association	www.nfauk.org
Nevus Outreach	www.nevus.org
Pemphigus Vulgaris Network	www.pemphigus.org.uk
Primary Immunodeficiency Association	www.pia.org.uk
Pseudoxanthoma Elasticum Support Group (PiXiE)	www.pxe.org.uk
Psoriasis Association	www.psoriasis-association.org.uk

Psoriasis & Psoriatic Arthritis Alliance	www.papaa.org
Restoration of Appearance and Function Trust	www.raft.ac.uk
Raynaud's & Scleroderma Association	www.raynauds.org.uk
Scleroderma Society	www.sclerodermasociety.co.uk
Shingles Support Society	www.shinglessupport.org
Skcin (Skin Cancer Information)	www.skcin.org
Skin Care Conditions Scotland	www.skinconditionscampaignscotland.org
Skin Care Cymru	www.skincarecymru.org
Skin Disorders A to Z	www.skindisordersatoz.com
Skinship UK	www.ukindex.info/skinship
Telangiectasia Self Help group	www.telangiectasia.co.uk
Terrence Higgins Trust	www.tht.org.uk
Tuberous Sclerosis Association	www.tuberous-sclerosis.org
Victim Support Group	www.victimsupport.co.uk
Vitiligo Society	www.vitiligosociety.org.uk
Wessex Cancer Trust	www.wessexcancer.org
Xeroderma Pigmentosum Support Group	www.xpsupportgroup.org.uk

CAMOUFLAGE PRODUCTS : those listed in bold capitals are available on GB NHS prescription and can be ordered directly from pharmacy counters as well as direct retail from the nominated supplier

Alida dePase Camouflage	Global – www.vitiligo-products.it
COVERMARK (Derma UK Ltd)	www.dermauk.co.uk
Coverderm Camouflage	Global - www.farmeco.com
DERMACOLOR (Kryolan)	UK - www.charlesfox.co.uk
	Global - www.kryolan.com
DERMABLEND Camouflage	UK – www.dermablend.co.uk
	Global www.dermablend.com
GloMinerals Camouflage	www.cle-europe.com
KEROMASK Camouflage	Global – www.bellava.co.uk
Jane Iredale Camouflage	Global - www.janeiredale.com
Supercover Camouflage	Global - www.beautyrepublica.com
VEIL (Thomas Blake Cosmetic Creams Ltd)	UK & Global – www.veilcovercream.com

The British Association of Skin Camouflage
www.skin-camouflage.net

recommended reading

All Party Parliamentary Group on Skin : London   Reports on,
The Enquiry into Fraudulent Practice in the treatment of Skin Disease (1999)
The Enquiry into the Impact of Skin diseases on People's Lives (2003)
Skin Cancer – Improving Prevention, Treatment and Care (2008)
Commissioning of Services for People with Skin Conditions (2008)

Dr Stephen & Gina Antczak (2001) *Cosmetics Unmasked*
Thorsons, London : ISBN 0 00 710568 1

Ashton, Richard and Leppard, Barbara (2005) *Differential Diagnosis in Dermatology*
Radcliffe Publishing Ltd, Oxon : ISBN 1 85775 660 6

Aucoin, Kevin (1997) *Making Faces*
Prion Books Ltd, London : ISBN 1 85375

Bates, B with Cleese, J (2001) *The Human Face*
BBC Worldwide Limited, London : ISBN 0 563 55188 7

Begoun, Paula (2003) *Don't Go To The Cosmetics Counter Without Me (8th edition)*
Beginning Press, Seattle WA, USA : ISBN 1 877988 30 8

Birren, Faber (1987) *The Principles of Colour*
Schiffer Publishing, Atglen, PA, USA :ISBN 0 88740 103 1

Etcoff, Nancy (2000) *Survival of the Prettiest, the science of beauty*
Abacus, London : ISBN 0 349 11048 0

Gawkrodger, David J (2002) *Dermatology, An Illustrated Colour Text (3rd Edition)*
Churchill Livingstone (Elsevier Science Ltd) : ISBN 0 443 07140 3

Gawkrodger, David J (2004) *Dermatology, Dermatology, A Rapid Reference*
Mosby (Elsevier Limited) : ISBN 0 7234   3379 8

Goffman, E (1963) *Stigma: Notes on the Management of Spoiled Identity*
Penguin Books, Harmondsworth : ISBN 13 978 0 671 62244 2

Grealy, L (1994) *In the Mind's Eye : an autobiography of a face*
Haughton Mifflin, New York : ISBN 1 85695 124 3

Goodman, Thomas and Young, Stephanie (1988) *Smart Face, a dermatologist's guide to saving your money and saving your skin*
Prentice Hall Press, New York, USA : ISBN 0 13 814377 3

Hull, Ruth (2009) *Anatomy & Physiology for beauty and complementary therapies*
The Write Idea, Cambridge : ISBN 01223 847765

Lansdown, R, Rumsey, N, Bradbury, E, Carr, A, Partridge, J. (Eds). (1997) *Visibly Different : Coping with Disfigurement.*
Butterworth Heinemann, London : ISBN 0 7506 3424 3

Lewis, Wendy (2001) *The Lowdown on Facelifts and Other Wrinkle Remedies*
Quadrille Publishing, London : ISBN 1 903845 25 4

Marks, R (2003) *Roxburgh's Common Skin Diseases (17th Edition)*
Arnold : Hodder Headline Group, London : ISBN 0 340 76232 2

E R Mayhew, ER (2004*) The Reconstruction of Warriors : Archibald McIndoe, the Royal Air Force and the Guinea Pig Club*
Greenhill Books, London : ISBN 1 85367 610 1

Dr Linda Papadopoulos (2005) *Mirror, Mirror*
Hodder & Stoughton, London : ISBN 0 340 83376 9

Papadopoulos, Linda and Bor, Robert (1997) *Psychological Approaches to Dermatology*
The British Psychological Society Books, Leicester : ISBN 1 85433 292 9

Papadopoulos Linda and Walker Carl (2003) *Understanding Skin Problems*
John Wiley & Sons Ltd, Chichester : ISBN 0 470 84518 X

Partridge, James (2012) *Changing Faces: the Challenge of Facial Disfigurement* (6th edition)
A Changing Faces publication, London   ISBN 978-1-900928-34-2

Pease, Allen, (1997) *Body Language – how to read others' thoughts by their gestures*
Sheldon Press London : ISBN 0 8555969 782 7

Piff, Christine (1985) *Let's Face It*
Victor Gollancz Ltd, London : ISBN 0 575 03533 1

Rumsey, Nichola and Harcourt, Diana (2005) *The Psychology of Appearance*
Open University Press, Maidenhead : ISBN 0 335 21276 X

Savona, Natalie and Holford, Patrick (2001) *Solve Your Skin Problems*
Judy Piatkus (Publishers) Ltd, London : ISBN 0 7499 2185 4

Smith, Virginia (2007) *Clean, a history of personal hygiene and purity*
Oxford University Press : ISBN 978 0 19 929779 5

Swami, Viren and Furnham, Adrian (2008) *The Psychology of Physical Attraction*
Routledge, Hove, East Sussex : ISBN 978 0 415 42251 2

Veale, David and Neziroglu, Fugen (2010) *Body Dysmorphic Disorder, a treatment manual*
Wiley-Blackwell, Chichester : ISBN 978 0 470 85121 0

Veale, David, Willson, Rob and Clarke Alex (2009) *Overcoming Body Image Problems, including Body Dysmorphic Disorder – a self-help guide using cognitive behavioural techniques.*
Constable & Robinson, London : ISBN 978 1 84529 279 9

White, Gary (2004) *Colour Atlas of Dermatology (3rd Edition)*
Mosby, Elsevier Science : ISBN 0 7234 3298 8

Winter, Ruth (2005) *Consumer's Dictionary of Cosmetic Ingredients (6th Edition)*
Three Rivers Press, New York : ISBN 1 4000 5233 5

Wolf, Naomi (1990) *The Beauty Myth*
Vintage Books, London : ISBN 0 09 986190 9

RESEARCH

Unfortunately, the efficacy (or not) of skin camouflage does not attracted much research. The following will aid your studies and references for articles; we accept this is not a definitive list as obviously there will other be studies which have not been brought to our attention.

All Party Parliamentary Group on Skin : Westminster, London. Reports on the Enquiry into the Impact of skin Diseases on People's Lives (2003) updated (2013)

Body image and disfigurement: issues and interventions. Rumsey N, Harcourt D. Centre for appearance Research.
Elsevier Body Image 1 (2004) 83-97

Cosmetic camouflage. C Antoniou, C Stefanaki.
Journal of Cosmetic Dermatology. (5) (2006) 297-301

Cosmetic camouflage advice improves quality of life. SA Holme, PE Beattie, CJ Fleming
Epidemiology and Health Services Research. British Journal Dermatology, Nov. 2002 : 147 846-949

Camouflage for patients with vitiligo vulgaris improved their quality of life. M Tanioka, Y Yamamoto, M Kato, Y Miyachi.
Journal of Cosmetic Dermatology (9 : 2010) 72-75

Emotional benefit of cosmetic camouflage in the treatment of facial skin conditions: personal experience and review. LL Levy, JJ Emer.
Clinical, Cosmetic & Investigational Dermatology (2012 : 5) 173-182

Evaluating the effectiveness of psychosocial interventions for individuals with visible differences: a systematic review of the empirical literature. A Bessell, TP Moss. Centre for Appearance Research.
Elsevier Body Image 4 (2007) 227-238

One in seven people with skin disease suffer silently with 'severe pain'
British Skin Foundation press release (2011)

Make-up improves the quality of life of acne patients without aggravating acne eruptions during treatments. Clinical Report
European Journal of Dermatology, Vol 15 No. 4 284-7 July-August 2005

Psychological and psychosocial functioning of children with burn scarring using cosmetic camouflage: a multi-centre prospective randomized controlled trial.
J Maskell, P Newcombe, G Martin, R Kimble.
Elsevier, Science Direct Burns 40 (2014) 135-149

Quality of Life in paediatric patients before and after cosmetic camouflage of visible skin conditions
ML Ramien, S Ondrejchak, R Gendron, A Hatami, CC McCuaig, J Powell, D Marcoux.
Journal of the American Academy of Dermatology July 2014

Quality of life and stigmatization profile in a cohort of vitiligo patients and effect of the use of camouflage. K Ongenae, L Dierckxsens, L Brochez, N van Geel, JM Nacyaert. Dermatology 2005

Skin Camouflage can help restore young people's self confidence
Elizabeth Allen
Dermatological Nursing, 2015 Vol 14 No 1 (18-23)

Skin Camouflage for the deceased
Elizabeth Allen
International Therapist issue 106 Oct 2013 (24-26)

Skin Conditions in the UK : Health Care Needs Assessment, J Schofield, D Gindlay, H Williams. Centre of Evidence based Dermatology, University of Nottingham.

Social Psychology of Facial Appearance (the) R Bull, N Rumsey. European Journal of Social Psychology, Vo. 24 issue 2 279-284 March-April 1994

cosmetic ingredients common to camouflage products

space does not allow us to include the ingredients found in *every* brand of skin camouflage, but as a guide we list those commonly used in the crèmes, setting powder fixing spray and mineral powder camouflage

ACRYLATES (Acrylates Copolymer)
are the salts, esters or conjugate bases of acrylic acid, used to thicken crèmes and possibly to make them feel more soft and spread easily.

ALCOHOLIA LANAE (lanolin alcohol) see lanolin

ALCOHOL DENAT(ured)
used as an anti-foaming astringent and antimicrobial. It is rendered unsuitable for drinking

ALCOHOL STYRAX BENZOIN (Storax or sweet oriental gum)
resin obtained from the bark, used as a weak antiseptic (benzoin is a UV absorber) – may cause allergic reaction

ANTIOXIDANTS
used to delay, or prevent, the fats and oils used in cosmetics/camouflage crèmes from becoming rancid

ALLANTOIN
colourless crystals used to help heal wounds and promote healthy tissue (synthetically prepared by heating uric acid with dichloroacetic acid or by the oxidation of uric acid)

ALUMINIUM HYDROXIDE
used as a skin protectant and opacifying agent (many sunscreens use it as a coating for titanium dioxide preventing it from clumping, and forms a refractive layer for UV rays

ASCORBYL PALMITATE
used as an antioxidant, synthetically obtained from ascorbic acid (vitamin c)

AQUA
sterile water – may be distilled or deionised – manufacturers may also need to remove/reduce high mineral content by water softening agents. Occasionally sea, mineral or spring water can be used, or special water such as from the Dead Sea

BEESWAX
usually yellow or bleached to white (for a more cosmetically acceptable preparation) the wax is obtained by melting the honeycomb of the bee and removing any impurities
- it raises congealing and melting point
- enables water to be incorporated in water-in-oil emulsions
note: hypersensitivity to beeswax has been reported

BENZOYL BENZOATE see paraben

BENZOPHENONE-3
used as fixative, soluble in most fixed oils and in mineral oil. Also used to help prevent deterioration of ingredients that might be affected by UV

BENZYL SALICATE (salicylic acid benzyl ester)
a thick liquid, with a pleasant smell used as a fixative in perfumes and as a solvent in sunscreen lotions. May cause skin rash when exposed to sunlight

BIS-HYDROXYPROPYL DIMETHICONE
a silicone oil, which acts as a wetting agent with moisturising and fragrance retention properties

BISMUTH OXYCHLORIDE
a grey-white powder with a bright metallic lustre, sometimes termed as "synthetic pearl" gives lustre to cosmetics

BLACKCURRANT (RIBES NIGRUM) SEED OIL
a vitamin rich oil known for skin, nail and hair strengthening properties

BP (B P) denotes ingredients conforms to **BRITISH PHARMACOPOEIA STANDARD**

BUTAN(E)
flammable, easily liquefiable gas derived from petroleum, used as a propellant for aerosol sprays often in conjunction with propane and isobutane (is an alternative to CFCs, which are known to damage the ozone layer)

BUTYL
derived from Butane

BUTYLATED HYDROXYANISOLE (BHA) and
BUTYLATED HYDROXYTOLUENE (BHT) (butylhydroxytoluol)

BHA yellow-white waxy solid, with aromatic odour used as an antioxidant in cosmetics, it delays or prevents rancidity of fats and oils

BHT antioxidant and preservative used in foods, beverages and cosmetics. A white crystalline solid (prohibited as a food additive in UK)

Caution: either may cause allergic reactions

BUTYLPARABEN
widely used in cosmetics as an antifungal preservative, the ester of butyl alcohol and p-hydroxybenzoic acid (one of a family of parabens widely used as antibacterial and antifungal)

CALCIUM CARBONATE
a chalk used as a dulling agent

CALCIUM SILICATE
a naturally occurring mineral and is a compound of calcium oxide and silicon dioxide; presents as a white free flowing powder, used as an anti-caking agent

CAMPHOR
preservative, moth repellent and used in the manufacture of lacquers and embalming fluid : from the tree Cinnamomum Camphora

CANDELILLA (WAX)
yellow-brown brittle lumps obtained from Candelillia plants, i.e. Eurphorbia (vegetable) wax produced in Mexico; used to harden other waxes and gives firmness to the product.

CARNAUBA WAX
made from the leaves of the Brazilian wax palm, a hard vegetable wax; gives firmness to the product, used as a hardener, raises melting point

CASTOR OIL
expressed from the seed of Palm Christi it is soothing to the skin : it forms a tough shiny film when dried

CERA ALBA see beeswax

CERAMICROCRISTALLINA (see Microcystaline Wax)

CETYL PEG/PPG-10/1 DIMETHICONE
one of the dimethicones used as a skin and hair conditioner; it is an emulsifier and prolongs the release of active molecules

CETYL PALMITATE
originally a white wax, obtained from whales - NO LONGER ALLOWED – now synthetically made from Palmitoyl Chloride and Cetyl Alcohol in the presence of Magnesium; used as a stabiliser

CITRIC ACID
a water soluble weak tri-basic acid found in many fruits, especially the citrus fruits (lemon juice contains 5-8%) also from pineapple waste; used as a preservative, also to enhance the effectiveness of anti-oxidants and as a mordant to brighten colours

COLOURING AGENTS
These fall into two groups, organic and inorganic (derived from minerals). The Colour Index (CI) is the nomenclature used to identify colouring agents used in EU products, whereas the US Food and Drug Administration (FDA) use their International Nomenclature for Cosmetic Ingredients (INCI) names. The following colours (prefix numbers = CI and suffix = USA Food, Drugs & Cosmetics use) are the ones most frequently used in cosmetics and toiletries,

12085	D&C red number 36	77163	bismuth chloride oxide : white (see individual entry)
15850	D&C red number 7	77266	carbon black
15850:1	D&C red number 7	77288	chromic oxide : green
15880	D&C red number 34	77289	chromium hydoxide : green
15985	FD&C yellow number 6	77491	iron oxide : red
15985:1	yellow lake	77492	FD & C yellow no 5
19140	D&C yellow number 5	77120	iron oxide : white 21
19140:1	yellow lake 5	77499	iron oxide : black
73015:1	food blue number 1	77510	ferric ferrocyanide : blue
75470	carmine of cochineal : red	77891	titanium dioxide : white (see individual entry)
77007	FD&C pigment blue	77947	zinc oxide : white
77077	ultra marine blue : blue 29		

COPOLYMER
a product derived from polymerisation of more than one species of monomer; prevents staining of colours

COUMARIN, CUMARIN (Tonka bean, Cumarin)
a fragrant ingredient taken from many plants, also made synthetically. Caution, may cause photosensitivity or allergic reaction

CYCLOPENTASILOXANE
used as a lubricant and solvent

DIMETHICONE
a white, viscous, silicone oil used to protect skin and as an ointment base ingredient

DISODIUM STEAROYL GLUTAMATE
used as a surfactant, moisturiser and consistency regulator

DISTEARDIMONIUM HECTORITE
used as a dispersing agent and to thicken oil based products and stabilise emulsions

ETHYL ALCOHOL (Ethanol)
used as a solvent, prepared by the fermentation of carbohydrates or synthetically from petroleum

ETHYLPARABEN
a preservative with antibacterial and antifungal properties, widely used in cosmetics

ETHYLHEXYL METHOXYCINNAMATE
used as a sunscreen in hypoallergenic cosmetics

FRAGRANCE and PERFUME (PARFUM)
fragrance additives are used to prevent the inconvenient smell from raw material dominating. In general, no camouflage cream "smells" of any fragrance or perfume, and is usually labelled as being either "fragrance" or "perfume free"

GLYCERIN (Glycerol)
used as a lubricating agent, humectant and improves smoothness

GLYCERYL STEARATE
a derivative of coconut oil, used as an aid for binding oil and water, i.e. a stabiliser of water-in-oil and oil-in-water emulsions; has emollient properties

HYDROGENATED POLYISOBUTENE
a synthetic oil used as a lubricant

IMIDAZOLIDINYL UREA
used as an antimicrobial and is a formaldehyde releasing preservative

IRON OXIDES
artificially made colours with high purity, used instead of natural iron oxides

ISOBUTYLPARABEN
widely used as a preservative (this ingredient is considered safe and used in cosmetics)

ISOPROPYL PALMITATE
widely used as a binder with emollient properties (research is on-going)

ISOPROPYL ALCOHOL
an antibacterial, solvent and denaturant prepared from propylene which is obtained in the cracking of petroleum

ISOPROPYL MYRISTATE
a synthetic oil used as a binding, also used as a solvent and as an emollient. Caution, comedogenic (undergoing review for continued and prolonged usage)

KAOLIN (China Clay)
extensively used in cosmetic powders because it has the ability to absorb sebum and moisture (insoluble in water) Caution, may clog the skin

LANOLIN (LANOLINE)
the "fat like" secretion of the sebaceous glands of sheep, which is deposited on the wool fibres. Lanolin contains approximately 25-30% water; pharmaceutically used as an ointment base and as a lubricant

LANOLIN ALCOHOL
solid waxy materials that are yellow to amber in colour, or pale to golden-yellow liquids derived from lanolin. Used as emulsifiers and emollients, less likely to cause allergic reactions than lanolin but may do so to sensitive skin

LAUROYL LYSINE
used as a binding agent, a surfactant and conditioning agent

LIMONENE
a synthetic flavouring agent used as a fragrance. Caution, a skin sensitiser and irritant

LINALOOL (Linalol)
used as a substitute for French lavender or bergamot; colourless liquid also used in food flavourings. May cause allergic reaction

LIQUID LANOLIN
viscous liquid derived from purified wool/fat sheep's wool, blends well with mineral and vegetable oils and is used as an emulsifying agent and emollient in skin creams; it is absorbed into the skin without the tackiness of wool fat, used as a mixing aid for binding oil and water

LIQUID PARAFFIN see MINERAL OIL, PARAFFIN & PETROLATUM

MAGNESIUM CARBONATE (also LIGHT MAGNESIUM CARBONATE)
organic salt, keeps powders light, used as a pressing aid; also used in tooth and face powders

MAGNESIUM MYRISTATE
magnesium salt of myristic acid (teradecanoic acid) which occurs (the acid) in nutmeg butter, and predominates in palm seed fats (20%) and occurs in most animal and vegetable fats; used as an adhering agent

MAGNESIUM SULFATE (Epsom Salts)
used for anti inflammatory properties

METHYLPARABEN
preservative : synthetic compound of the benzoate family

MICA
mainly used as a colouring (pale green, brown or black to colourless) and to give a glow to the product. Also used as a lubricant

MICROCRYSTALLINE WAX
any of various plastic materials obtained from petroleum; they differ from paraffin waxes in that they have a higher melting point, higher viscosity and much finer (micro) crystals

MINERAL OIL also see Paraffin & Petrolatum
light mineral oil = light liquid paraffin
white mineral oil = liquid paraffin
purified oil of mineral origin, e.g. petroleum (Canadian = liquid paraffin) used to improve textures, stability or water repellent properties of final preparation; uses - emulsifying and emollient properties, as a lubricant

NYLON-12
used to opacify and thicken

OCTYLDODENCANOL
derivative of coconut oil, an oil with good mixing qualities; used as a spreading agent, has good mixing properties; used for binding powders

OLETH 10 (BRAND NAME) OLEYL ALCOHOL
found in fish oils, chiefly used in the production of detergents and wetting agents, also an anti-foam agent and plasticiser; used as an emulsion stabiliser and skin emollient
note multi ingredient preparation containing Oleyl Alcohol is Polytar & Polytar Plus

OZOKERITE see CERESIN WAX / MICROCRYSTALLINE WAX

PARABEN (suffix) methyl- propyl- and parahydroxybenzoate are the most common
a little group of **Hydroxybenzoates** : widely used, estimated to be found in 75-90% of all cosmetics and toiletries : they are preservatives with antibacterial and anti-fungal properties.
In 2004 a study published in the Journal of Applied Toxicology reported that parabens are a cause for concern, and are believed to act like the female hormone oestrogen (high levels of oestrogen can cause some women to develop breast cancer). research is ongoing

PARAFFIN, PARAFFIN WAX
alkaline hydrocarbons, purified wax from mineral oil; hard paraffin : liquid paraffin :
white   soft paraffin : yellow soft paraffin : light liquid paraffin
are all used as bases for the preparation of creams, and to thicken products which raises the melting point and stability; also used as a solvent   see Mineral Oil

PARAFFINUM LIQUIDUM see LIQUID PARAFFIN

PERFUME see Fragrance

PETROLATUM (petroleum jelly, paraffin jelly)
used for its emollient properties, it is almost insoluble in water, found in most cosmetic products. Helps to soften the skin, prevents evaporation of moisture from the skin and acts as a protector against irritations. Although generally non-toxic it has been found to cause allergic reactions.

PHENOXYETHANOL
widely used as a bactericide and as a topical antiseptic; it has a faint aromatic odour which can be used to perfume cosmetics

POLYBUTENE
a polymer obtained from petroleum oils used to lubricate

POLYGLYCERYL-4 ISOLSTEARATE
used as an emulsifier and stabilise

PROPANE
used as an aerating ingredient in cosmetics and as a propellant in aerosols

PROPYLENE GLYCOL
hygroscopic, viscous liquid, used as a non-toxic anti-freeze in breweries and dairies, it inhibits fermentation and mould growth in products; used in the manufacture of synthetic resins

PROPYLPARABEN
an artificial hard wax, which raises melting point; as a preservative they have antibacterial and anti-fungal properties; widely used in cosmetics in concentrations up to 0.1%

PROPYL GALLATE, PROPYLIS GALLAS, PROPYLUM GALLICUM
presents as a white powder, has antioxidant properties when used in cosmetics and foods; prevents the deterioration and rancidity of fats and oils

SILICA
a white powder (such as sand) used for colour and for its absorbent properties

SODIUM CARBONATE (soda ash)
odourless small crystals that occur in ores, seawater and lake brines. Absorbs water from the air

SORBITOL
similar to, but less expensive, than naturally occurring glycerin. A common ingredient used as a humectant (leaves skin with a soft, velvety feel.) Derived from seaweed, algae, and fruits or by chemical reduction of glucose.

STEARYL STEARATE
used as an emulsifier, emollient and thickener

TALC
White/grey/brown/pale green mineral - talcum – hydrated magnesium silicate, purified French chalk = Talcum Purificatum. Used as a fine powder, used for colouring matter, also to spread make-up on the skin; it adheres readily to the skin, when used in dusting powders it should be sterilised

TITANIUM DIOXIDE also called Titanium Oxide, Titanic Oxide, Titanium Dioxide Coated Mica, Titanium Dioxide CI.77891
white insoluble powder occurring naturally as a mineral and used chiefly as a pigment of high covering power and durability that also reflects UV light and is used as a natural protection against the sun

caution, can cause "flash back white" on photographs taken indoors and with the flash facility activated and may "grey" and dull the skin to skin groups 4 5 & 6 (and to 1 2 & 3 with a natural sheen)

TOCOPHEROL
a preservative which prevents rancidity; pharmaceutically Tocopherol is usually prefixed œ or Alpha, and is Vitamin E which is a fat-soluble vitamin. It is found in preparations such as evening primrose oil capsules. It may well oxidise when added to BHT and hereby acting as a preservative, just like vitamin C (Ascorbic Acid). also see BHT

UREA
colourless crystals, very soluble in water, used extensively in cosmetics and toiletries as an antiseptic, deodoriser, humectant and antimicrobial preservative (uric acid is used as a skin conditioner)
Note, urea can be excreted from (human) urine but is usually prepared synthetically

ZINC STEARATE (ZINCI STEARAS)
used as a lubricant, an artificially made powder from stearic acid and palm oil, a white amorphous powder which is insoluble - a good soft powder with good adhesion - used alone, or with other powders, or in the form of a cream

GLOSSARY OF TERMINOLOGY USED

"beauty therapist" includes qualified:
- beauty aesthetician
- holistic therapist

"medical adviser" includes qualified:
- doctor-consultant
- maxillofacial technician
- nurse
- occupational therapist
- pharmacist

dermatosis
- medical skin condition

erythema
- red

lesion
- area of skin different to surrounding skin

hyper
- extra, more than

hypo
- none, less than

the **B**ritish **A**ssociation of **S**kin **C**amouflage (founded in 1985) is an independent, non-profit making charity, which is not affiliated to any industry, company, organisation or authority. We only link our name and logo to that which we believe to be beneficial to our objective.

Our objective is to alleviate the psychological, physical and social effects that an "altered" image can have on people's lives by the simple application of specialised products.

We do not endorse or sell products.
We consider that such action allows us to work in a non-biased way
which is free from another's influence or agenda.

We are dedicated to providing a skin camouflage service for men, women and children of all ages, regardless of ethnicity or religion.

Anyone can take advantage of the skin camouflage service
provided by BASC trained professionals within the NHS and private practice.

BASC Associate Membership is open to any group, person
and organisation interested in skin camouflage.

We continually campaign for a better understanding of the psychological
and social-economical problems associated with an image that
may be considered different to others.

BASC is acknowledged as the leading provider for training
medical professionals, maxillofacial technicians, pharmacists,
make-up artists, therapists and tutors equipping them with the skills necessary to
undertake hospital, clinic, salon and college practice.

BASC is run by professionals who volunteer their expertise.
Our trained consultants work independently of BASC – we do not employ any staff.

We continue to review our activities and consult with
Patient Support Groups and medical organisations in order to improve
the camouflage provision available and
to ensure it is appropriate for people in the 21st Century

further information concerning the Association and training opportunities
can be found on our website
www.skin-camouflage.net

Lightning Source UK Ltd.
Milton Keynes UK
UKIC01n0943140815
256926UK00014B/34

9 781452 066035